Make the Shift

A Proven Method
for Busy Professionals
to Transform Their Health,
Wellbeing and Confidence

Serena Sabala

Published by

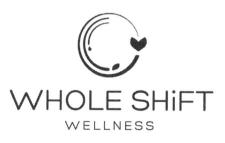

WHOLE SHiFT
WELLNESS

Dear Robby,

Thank you for your very inspiring work. You guys are changing lives in a radical way. I am inspired by what you stand for. Here is a token from me to you. Enjoy and hope to meet you both in person soon.

Serena

ISBN: 9781711095103

Make the Shift reviews

"*I fall into the stereotype of the entrepreneur charging forward in pursuit of a goal, sacrificing everything to do good by others, but in the process placing my own wellbeing at the bottom of the pile. Of course, I won't admit this to myself or others, but Serena's book creates an environment where I feel ok to be honest with my body. She's not judging, nor preaching; she's bringing me with her – encouraging me to adopt measured changes that shift my thinking towards my own health. Serena humanises the wellbeing narrative. Her book explores scientific fact, without imposing it on you, leaving you to explore her ideas for yourself. She splices accessible tips and minor innovations we can all adopt to improve our everyday lives. I now start my day with a litre of water and my soul also feels lighter now I have shifted more towards a plant-based diet.*

"*Serena's words come from a deep rooted instinct to help people find their inner love. Her words have had a profound impact on my state of mind. I feel that I am now on a different course where I now know that I will only achieve my goals if I put my wellbeing first.*"

Stephen Willard – Founder, EMBLAZE

"*The Whole Shift Method is a long overdue breath of fresh air within the health and wellness space. It's easy for any highly-driven person to be vulnerable to the high-intensity 'quick fixes' so well-represented by the wellness industry, and that's because it makes desirable promises. However many savvy professionals are ready to acknowledge that it's the compounding effect of smaller actions which are necessary to create real and lasting change. The Whole Shift Method takes all of the guessing out of what those actions are and how to easily apply them*".

Lydia McCarthy-Keen Keen, luxury jeweller,
ethical engagement ring specialist, and the UKs
leading expert on lab-grown diamonds.

"The Whole Shift Approach is a game-changer for busy entrepreneurs who need to consistently step their game up, live outside of their comfort zone while trying to maintain their health. One of the biggest challenges entrepreneurs face is 'balance', the balance of mind, body, emotion, focus and that's exactly what Serena and the Whole Shift Approach solves. Serena's long term, holistic approach will dive deep into a methodology that will help you make a bigger impact, live a healthier life, have more fun and most importantly, do it all for longer!"

Sebastian Bates, Best Selling Author
and Founder of the Global Warrior Academy

"Being an entrepreneur I am guilty of often sacrificing my health & wellbeing for the sake of moving my business forward. And like many of us I have always had the inner voice telling me that something had to change if I was to take my business to the next level and stay in the game for the long run. After reading this book I was left feeling that I have finally received a step-by-step guide on how to love myself better both my body & mind, and how to transform my mindset to make a lasting change.

"The book is deeply personal and the real life examples create many AHA moments. It is also very practical – almost like a manual of how not to sabotage your best intentions of living healthier & more sustainably. Like an expert coach Serena helps the readers to discover their blind spots and their limiting beliefs and then empowers them to make a shift and rediscover the greatness within. It is a great read for everyone that wants to take a wholistic approach on changing their lifestyle from "good enough" to "great". This book should be on every CEO's "must read list". I cannot recommend it highly enough!"

Andra Raju – Founder, Inspiriko

"What a joy to read such a complete book. A book that gives clear counsel on how to achieve the three critical pillars of health and wellbeing; focus, food and fitness – and to my mind valued direction to execute physical performance improvement. As an Ironman triathlete and business owner, I require strong focus in both of my passionate worlds, but the reality is... life gets in the way! Serena's well-defined methodology has allowed me to overcome many of the eating hurdles I have when working long hours and exercising. Serena aptly calls this wonderful transformation, #makingtheshift. Personally this is a shift to a more successful entrepreneur, stronger athlete and mother & wife with more energy! Thank you Serena."

Cara Cunniff – Founder,
Property Precision – Endurance Athlete

"When we want to achieve long lasting results at anything, it is so important to adopt the right mindset.

"If we want to lose weight, be vibrant and healthy, people think that it's simply a case of eating healthy and exercising. But if it were that simple, we would be a far more healthier nation and planet.

"Being a speculative investor, I can appreciate that success is not necessarily linked purely to skill either. Instead, it is the mindset of developing a consistent plan and sticking to it.

"What I love about Serena and Wholeshift Wellness is their ability to break down goals for each individual making it not only easy to achieve, but to be liberating, long lasting and sustainable.

"Serena and her team aren't just helping people achieve their health goals, they are helping people understand how to make long-lasting and sustainable changes for themselves and their loved ones.

"Amazing read."

Jason Graystone – Investor, Entrepreneur –
Founder, Tiers of Freedom. Graystone Education Ltd

"Serena Sabala's book changes perspectives. Many of us think that maintaining a healthy lifestyle is challenging. Dieting and eating healthy is considered a deprivation, and eating "naughty" food is rather seen as indulgent and a reward. Serena explains in a very simple and logical way how our perception of food and health is dictated by our mindset. She proves that it is possible to change that mindset and also gives us the tools to achieve it. The book is a page-turner and it will make you reconsider your views about your most valuable asset – your health."

Michaela Hardt – Founder, Nutmad

"Serena Sabala is a passionate health and wellness expert, she's worked for ten years in five countries, and from her insights, she has distilled a profound methodology that we can read and implement immediately. In the Whole Shift Approach, she highlights common obstacles and pitfalls and gives step-by-step guidance and direction to enable us to take control of our health and wellness journey. I found it so compelling on my first read that I applied the Focus methodology before I finished the book and the results are transformative and have crossed over into all areas of my life and my creative practice."

Paula Barnard-Groves Artist – Founder, Sculptor43

"The Whole Shift Approach moves beyond traditional boundaries to recognise the importance of harmonising the mind with the body in order to create lasting change. Serena Sabala simultaneously provides clarity and addresses common misconceptions about health and wellbeing to provide a crucial roadmap to enduring results. Using a holistic lens, The Whole Shift Approach provides a comprehensive toolkit to help you make the shift."

Dr. Jonathan Ashong-Lamptey –
Host of The Element of Inclusion

"The best way to change your life is to change what your life is made up of--your rituals, your habits, how you eat and think and the Whole Shift Approach is a road map for doing exactly that. Written by Serena Sabala — this handbook is a refreshing, insightful and practical guide for busy entrepreneurs looking to maintain peak levels of health and well-being over the long-term, with proven methodologies to achieve that from her years of experience helping other entrepreneurs to do the same."

Robyn Ford – Founder, The Wild Together

"If you think this book is only another one on "how-to" lose weight, or "how-to" be fit, think again! This is a precious guide, a bright resource to become the best version of ourselves; It is an invitation to reflect on our patterns, actions and results that we are getting from them. Serena's methodology encourages us to take a holistic approach to recognize and explore our habits, and tackle what is getting in the way of our greatest potential.

"I am still dipping my toes into the literacy of health and wellness and how to improve my wellbeing, finding what works for me and what doesn't, but in Serena's words I found comfort, I found motivation and the structure to make long lasting life changes. It is an invitation to look *for excellence using a powerful methodology which has never been expressed with such intensity, passion and empowerment. It shows the way to be our best selves and find balance in all area of our lives."*

Leticia Dolenga – Founder, Mesh Hub

"A "must read". The Whole Shift Method offers more than sound advice and coaching on nutrition. Serena Sabala understands and communicates the importance of recognizing we are more than just a body. Her sage advice and fair warnings guide us through the obstacles , and how to overcome them, that are sure to arise when we set out on the journey to a healthy lifestyle. Whole Shift Method helps you take the wheel with confidence and inspires you to believe in your own ability to live your best healthy life. For anyone looking for guidance and clarity in navigating the confusing world of wellness and nutrition I highly recommend you read this book. Serena's ability to filter otherwise difficult concepts in an easy to understand way will surely help you believe that you can take the reins in caring for your most important asset – You."

Stacey Stier - Owner, Bikram Yoga North Texas

"Serena in her past and her present has seen firsthand the intensity of entrepreneurial stress. Her fluid book full of tips and exercises to make you think are helpful to creating a nurturing core of behaviours."

Mallika Paulraj – Author, "How The Best Invest"

Dedication

This book is dedicated to you. Yes that's right you, who picked it up and are choosing to invest your time in reading it: time is the most precious commodity we have in this world so I don't take this for granted and I thank you for it. I dedicate this book to you and everyone else who, like you, is choosing every day to make the time for learning new ways to improve their health, wellbeing and mind-body confidence. I know it is often not the easy thing to do and I applaud you for taking one step in the right direction by choosing to read this book.

I hope it will inspire you to never settle and give up on yourself because life is precious and it's never too late to get started living it to its fullest!

Contents

CHAPTER 1

Introduction

About love

The title of this book may lead you to think that this is a book about fitness or nutrition: full of tips on what exercises to do to get more lean and fit. You're probably hoping to get some recipes and meal plans to get you started with healthy eating. Who knows, you may even be expecting to discover some "secrets" that will finally make a huge difference to your wellness journey and get you the results you're hoping to achieve.

Let me break it to you: this book is, before anything else, a book about Love.

When I say Love, I'm not referring to the romantic kind of Love that first springs to mind. I'm talking about what we believe to be the most powerful force in the Universe: what makes us who we are and motivates us at the deepest level. That which brings us together and brings out the best in us through life. That's the Love I'm talking about. And let me tell you, that kind of Love has A LOT to do with your health and wellbeing. More than you can imagine.

And yes, you will also get a lot of invaluable information that specifically pertain to wellness: I intend to exceed your expectations so don't be alarmed! But what I feel sets us apart from any other approach to health and wellbeing is that we will get you to dig deep to the roots of your roadblocks and obstacles, so that whatever new results you achieve can be yours for life. You won't simply be doing things differently for a while, you will actually transform your habits and motivation from deep within. Our aim is not merely to change what you do and how: it is to change why.

Of course there will be ups and downs along the way, I'd be lying to you if I said otherwise. But you will never go back to the way things were, simply because you won't be that person any longer.

> Having said all that, I'd like to start with a powerful exercise. Please don't read on before you've completed it. This is so that you can get the greatest possible benefit from it.
>
> So put pen to paper and please write down below who you deem to be the most important person in your life: who do you love the most? Whose needs do you put first above anyone else's? Who do you cherish the most and take greatest care of each and every day?
>
> I know this is a tricky question, especially if you have more than one child as no parent can ever choose one child above the others so I'll make an exception for you and allow you to write them all down, but that aside, I invite you to choose one person above anyone else.
>
> _____

Well done for making this tough choice! I know how hard it can be to choose just one person but I firmly believe we ALL have that one special individual who has the power to make everything better (or worse), who can fill you with joy within seconds; the person who most often has solutions for our greatest questions and doubts. The person that can keep you motivated when things get tough. The person that can make you feel loved and cared for even when nobody else is around. That special person that is most deserving of your unconditional love, attention and care every single day because as long as they are cared for fully and completely, then you know all will be well in the end.

So keep that person's name in mind and trust me when I say that this exercise will make more sense in a little bit.

Let's delve deeper now, starting from what the "Whole Shift" method is all about and how it was born. I truly hope you enjoy the ride.

To keep in touch with the author, simply visit www.wholeshiftwellness.com

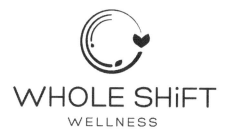

WHOLE SHiFT
WELLNESS

CHAPTER 2

The Whole Shift Method

Why I do what I do

One of the greatest obstacles that professionals face when trying to improve their level of fitness and wellbeing, is time. Really, if I had a pound for every time someone told me they just "don't have time" to improve their wellness routines …well let's say I'd be buying WAY more Stella McCartney bags than I currently do! This issue feels particularly insurmountable to parent of small children: in many cases it really is the "make or break" factor in determining whether someone will indeed take action towards shifting their habits for the better.

Now let me tell you a story: my story, actually, and my father's story. You see, after spending hours (and I mean HOURS) researching and investigation my purpose and our company's mission statement, I realized just how far back the seed was planted for me to become who I am and do what I do.

My dad was a VERY successful entrepreneur. In his early thirties, he quit his safe full time job to start a business whose revenue he grew to several millions euros in under 10 years. He actually invented a profession that didn't really exist before his time.

He was brilliant, successful, wealthy and had it all, or so it seemed. Until he lost it all. When I was only 8 years old my dad became ill and was diagnosed with Bipolar Disorder, a mental illness which is a trickier variation of depression. Anyone who has ever had anything to do with Bipolar, whether directly or indirectly, knows what a truly invasive and difficult illness it is.

What followed were far and away the most challenging years of my life, and my dad's illness remains to this day the hardest thing I've ever had to overcome. Now I feel that while I'm lucky to have had the strength (also thanks to my amazing and supportive family) to turn it into a formative experience, and I embrace it fully for making me who I am, I wouldn't wish the same childhood on anyone else. I know that many are not as lucky as I was and end up completely derailed after growing up in such a dysfunctional environment.

I see now with great clarity that my dad simply didn't have the tools to handle the mounting pressure of a highly demanding creative job and running a business on his own, whilst also doing his best to care for a young family. He literally crumbled under the pressure and lost EVERYTHING he had worked so hard to achieve over many years and sadly has never quite recovered since. These experiences are what planted the seed of wellness in me at such a young age: very early on I started to investigate ways that I could become a stronger and healthier version of myself, physically and emotionally and I haven't finished yet!

The consequences of my dad's diagnosis were profound and traumatizing not only to him but also us and ALL the many communities around him. Our entire family had to deal with many issues from financial to medical, all his 15+ employees lost their jobs quite unexpectedly, clients and work associates lost an amazing supplier and colleague who was truly hard to replace.

I often share this story with our clients who are struggling to prioritize their own self-care. I also tell them (and I truly believe this wholeheartedly) that if my dad had had the courage and strength to take months or even years off from his life and responsibilities to focus exclusively on his wellbeing and recovery, all of us would have had such a better life for it. Not to mention how much suffering and loss could have been prevented if he'd had the wisdom to realize he needed help and time for himself BEFORE he got ill. I would have gladly traded hours of his time and all the fancy clothes, cars and trips for a healthy father who could have been there for me physically and emotionally as I grew up. The problem is that he wasn't willing to make this trade himself: he gave more importance to his worldly success than his health which sadly led to him losing both.

We often think of our fitness and wellbeing routines as something we do "just for us" but the truth is, it's not just for us.

When we're strong, fit, healthy and fully satisfied, we go through life with different energy and stamina; we have more to contribute and generally do a better job all around. This extends far beyond the workplace too: we are better care takers, parents, friends and partners. We're happier in our body and mind and therefore are more pleasant to be around. Not to mention, and this is huge for young parents in particular, we are a great example to our kids who will inevitably pick up the good habits, consciously or unconsciously (instead of having to learn them the hard way, like I did.)

So next time you struggle to make time for a run, nap, massage or to cook yourself a healthy meal because "the kids come first" – think again. Your kids want nothing more than for you to be your healthiest, fittest, happiest and most satisfied self because if you're not, they can't be either. It really is that simple.

So now, let's go back to the exercise we did in the previous chapter and let me ask the same question again: who is the most important person in your life?

I hope you're now thinking what I'm thinking: YOU should be your first love and number one priority. YOU are the one that can make it all better.

Only if you love yourself first and fully, can you then love somebody else fully (and yes, that includes your children and parents.)

Only if you take care of yourself every single day, will you have the energy needed to take care of others.

There is no way around this.

So today and every day, we invite you to look in the mirror and acknowledge and be ready to love yourself more than anyone else, so that you can then go out into the world with an overflow of Love to offer to those around you.

Taking care of ourselves should be your top priority, because if we don't, soon enough somebody else will have to; and if you have children, it may just end up being them. I know often times it's easier said than done and essentially, that's why I do what I do.

I want to empower as many business owners and CEOs as I can to establish solid, sustainable wellness routines in their daily habits so that none of them will ever have to face the traumas my family and I went through.

Don't believe anyone who tells you it's not possible. Don't settle for "good enough". Don't wait until things get a little easier as it's likely they'll never do. Most importantly, don't use your kids as an excuse: use them as a motivation to make it even more of a priority. Start now. #maketheshift

Our Values

I was recently asked to distill what we do, here at Whole Shift Wellness, into three core values and I must say what felt like a simple exercise turned out to be an incredibly profound experience.

We often go about life thinking that we are clear on our values, assuming that we know what matters most to us and why. How often do we actually take the time to explore this subject though? The answer is probably not often enough.

I believe we often fail to leverage on our values for two main reasons.

The first one is that we don't take ownership over values: we think they're somewhat pre-determined and just accept them for what they are. For sure some values are deeply embedded since childhood; some of them are probably our parents' values that they passed onto us and we simply grew up believing them and not questioning them. The thing is, your values shape your life. So if you're living by someone else's values, you're essentially living according to someone else's rules.

You want to know what you value most in life? Well that's simple, what do you spend most money on?

Now, let's take some time for another "pen to paper" exercise: please write down your five most precious possessions and their rough monetary value. We don't need an exact amount so don't bother spending hours on some real estate website trying to figure out the current market value of your home. just a rough estimate will do, or the price you paid for it when you bought it, but make sure you list the top five and put down an actual figure rather than a range:

1.
2.
3.
4.
5.

And now list the five items that you spend most money each month on "maintaining". Chances are that most items will overlap with the above list but they may not (i.e. you may have spent a lot of money on your house but you may be spending more money each month on the maintenance and upkeep of your car or vice versa.)

1.
2.
3.
4.
5.

Now let me ask you another question: How much do you think your body is worth? if you were to give it a monetary value, how much would that be?

_____

If somebody came to you tomorrow and told you that you need a new body at all costs, would you trade in any of your prized possessions for it? My guess is that you would. In fact you probably would trade them all if you had to! And sadly many people every day end up doing just that: they spend their entire adult lives neglecting their health and wellbeing just for the sake of making money and when their bodies give up on them, they end up spending a fortune trying to regain their lost health.

Prevention is ALWAYS the most effective, cheapest and quickest cure, hands down, so every time you "cut down" on expenses or time pertaining to maintaining your health and wellbeing, you may just be doing yourself a huge disservice in the long run. The beautiful thing is that once you establish a solid foundation, maintaining a healthy and thriving Mind-Body will become a lot cheaper and it will pay HUGE dividends in longevity and vitality in the long run.

Take a moment to analyze this list and see if "you're putting your money where your mouth is": do these items match what you say you value most in life or can you notice any dissonance? I know what you may be thinking right now: the market value of certain items is simply higher that other things so you have no choice than to be spending more money on those. That is certainly true, but only to a point. I'll give you a practical example: we're currently living in an inexpensive rental property in an area of town that is not very central and not particularly nice. Sure, we could move somewhere nicer and more affluent, however we're choosing to stay put so that we can continue to invest money in our growing business. So we're valuing our business more than we're valuing where we live. We also spend more money on food than possibly anything else each month other than rent: that is because eating the healthiest, highest quality organic food is very high on our values and I would cut down on a lot of things before I cut down on that.

I spend what some people would deem to be an outrageous amount of money on an online workout streaming program: those same people however may be spending that much, or more, on going out for drinks and dinners each month.

I'm using these as examples of how to really assess what you currently value most so you can then identify if the list is coherent to you: do the above items match what you say you value most? Do they match your greatest goals and aspirations or are they a reflection of outdated values and priorities? Take a moment to have a look, think about this and write down any thoughts and considerations that come to mind.

The second reason why we lose power over our values, is that we feel they're set in stone therefore once acquired, they should never change. We end up identifying with them. We feel they're us and therefore resist changing them for fear that we may "lose ourselves".

Well I have good news for you: you are not your values.

You have a car, but you're certainly not a car. You have a house, but you're not a house either. Your house may shape your life because it affects where and how you spend time, the people you see, the activities you have access to but at some point you may find that you need more space or you want to experience different places, people and activities and therefore you move house. The same principle applies to your values. It may feel a little daunting to change your values, much as it can feel a little daunting to move house, but if you're looking to grow and expand, you can't avoid it.

Time and time again we see busy and time pressed professionals struggle to achieve their wellness goals: they keep prioritizing everything but the very actions they need to take in order to improve. This is simply because they don't go through the process of assessing and re-shaping their values.

They talk the talk but don't put their money where their mouth is: they keep spending money on expensive technology and trips to the pub, rather than healthy meal deliveries and a personal trainer.

So now, list the goals and objectives that you want to achieve in the next 3-5 years and see how you need to upgrade the above lists in order to manifest those things. What actions do you need to start spending more time, money and energy on, in order to get there?

And just for inspiration, let me share with you the values that drive our actions here at Whole Shift Wellness.

Be Selfish. We believe that YOU are the most important person in your life so you MUST take care of yourself first.

Be Selfless. We believe that the more YOU have, the more you have to GIVE. So be your best in order to be able to give your best.

Play big. We believe that you are capable of WAY more than you think you are. So don't hold back, the world deserves nothing less than you achieving your full potential.

So now, let me ask you, what do YOU believe? **#maketheshift**

IMPORTANT NOTE

The purpose of this book is to inspire, motivate and support you on the journey to your most fit, healthy and confident self. All the information I'll share is based not only on my personal experience but also on our work which spans over 20+ years combined, across 5 countries. I would however encourage you to consult a physician before making any changes to your health and wellness habits; please always bare in mind your own unique circumstances and current level of fitness and wellbeing, when taking on any new activities.

Wholistic Wellness: an industry trend that's here to stay

We are not lacking in trends these days: every day a new take on wellbeing arrives, and claims start rolling in of how revolutionary this new yoga class, superfood, supplement or approach is, and how it will transform your life. We expect them around every corner and, since it's virtually impossible at first glance to distinguish the fads from the facts, most of us have embraced a slightly detached and cynical approach to all of them.

I've studied nutrition for over 10 years now and even I find it hard to navigate the world of information these days. Even when a claim is supposedly backed by scientific research, it doesn't guarantee that it will be sound science, rather than a study designed or summarized in a biased way to support a hidden agenda. After all, pharmaceutical companies, food companies, supplement companies and even gurus and experts are all out there to earn a living, so we would be naive to expect an objective perspective from all of them.

Not to mention that even professionals and doctors are human beings with their own biases and limitations that may influence their recommendations.

The problem with science these days is that it is so obsessively focused on the smallest possible details, that it often fails to address the big picture. Just think about it: we have doctors who are specialized in the smallest organ, body part, cell, DNA strand or function of the body. We've been trained to believe that if we want to resolve an ailment of any sort, we must see the best specialist in that very specific field. The more specialized his knowledge, the better.

We've done the same with nutritional science and food in general: hardly anybody talks about food anymore. They all seem to talk about nutrients (did I get enough protein? are carbs bad for us? does sugar cause disease?) or functions (what about insulin resistance? is ketosis the way forward?).

I want to clarify that I don't have anything against traditional science and its advancement: I think it is impressive how far we've come and how effectively we can operate on the human body.

The question that comes to mind however is: why is it that we're more advanced than ever in the scientific field yet we're also more overweight and sick than ever before and progressively getting worse? Apparently, this newest generation of children will be the first to have a lower life expectancy than their parents: can you believe that?

It is virtually impossible for anyone in their everyday life to go through each piece of information in detail and understand scientific studies and claims in a way that will allow them to discern what's true from what's not and let's be fair, information agencies like BIG news more than they like the truth.

In all this madness, I've found the best approach is actually the very opposite of what we're often encouraged to do: and that is to take several steps back and try to regain a sense of the bigger picture.

Perhaps getting so laser-beam focused on tiny little details is distracting us from the big picture? My meditation teacher often tells the story of the three blind man that are put next to an elephant and asked to touch it and describe what an elephant is. One of the men happens to touch the tail of the elephant so he righteously claims "an elephant is like a tight rope that goes in circles", the next man touches a leg of the elephant and says "an elephant is like the large trunk of a solid tree", finally the last man happens to touch the trunk of the elephant and claims "an elephant is like a big snake that floats in the air". Were any of these men wrong? Not at all. They were all describing A PART of the elephant correctly. None of them however captured the full picture of what a whole elephant looks like.

The conclusion therefore should be, when we approach wellbeing, we should be thinking of us as a whole, how to take care of all aspects that make us who we are in an effort to bring balance. Doing just a lot of one thing (even if it's the right thing) is not the answer but making small incremental improvements across the three main pillars of wellbeing, as we've identified them will bring forth exponential improvements.

The same goes with food: let's shift the focus out of individual nutrients and back to the foods that are commonly known and recognized by most diets as being conducive to our optimal wellbeing. Most schools of nutrition (other than those that are very extreme) will agree on general points so if you want to make some improvements, start from those points: eat more fruit and vegetables (5 of more helpings of each category a day), favor wholegrain and legumes instead of refined carbohydrates, avoid junk food, processed food and fizzy drinks, limit the consumption of alcohol and sugary/fatty treats.

Confusion and overwhelm are the enemy of implementation so take a step back, look at the big picture and use your common sense to start from the obvious improvements you ALREADY know you should be making; then once you've tackled what you can on your own, perhaps consider working with a specialist to get more specific advice but ALWAYS remember to take a step back every so often and look at the big picture.

I firmly believe that a wholistic approach to wellbeing is not just a fad or fancy trend. It's a fundamental evolutionary step we MUST take as a species if we want to not only survive, but thrive in life. I'm not a massive fan of sensationalism but I have absolutely no doubt that humanity is at the cusp of a major shift in consciousness: one that has the potential to see us take a massive step backwards if we deny the truth of our condition. However, if we choose to face our reality, as harsh as it may be, and learn from our previous mistaken approaches, we will take a huge leap forward into a beautiful next phase. I don't know about you, but that's what I'm working for!

A Powerful Junction: Why Wellness and Sustainability go hand in hand

We always say to our Shifters: "Your body is the Ferrari you drive through life" and by now it should be clear what we mean by that. If you had a Ferrari (or even if you do!), would you get the cheapest oil and fuel for it, or go out of your way to find the highest quality the market has to offer? Would you trash it daily, leave litter inside it and take poor care of it? Or would you take extra care to maintain its pristine state and immediately clean it if it gets dirty?

Every time you trash your body, every time you neglect it, every time you feed it trashy foods and drinks and fail to maintain it the way it deserves to, you're effectively trashing something that has a monetary value that's WAY greater than a Ferrari, we've now firmly established that.

And much as the body is the Ferrari we drive through life, Plane Earth is the home we are so lucky to inhabit during this life. How much is this beautiful planet worth? All the money in the world would not be enough to buy a new one if this breaks down for good.

That's why we believe that magic happens at the junction between wellness and sustainability. The moment you take a step back and look at everything from a grander perspective, you will start realizing what the things are that really matter most in this life and re-shuffle all your priorities around your newfound greater perspective. This will inevitably have a profound positive effect, not only on your health and wellbeing, but it will also create a ripple effect of positive transformation throughout all areas of your life because guess what: everything is closely linked and interconnected. Life is not a house with lots of different rooms behind closed doors: it is more like open plan living with hardly any walls to separate one space from another. What you do in one area, will inevitably have an effect on all other areas to some extent.

By appreciating the insurmountable value of your Mind and Body, your precious Ferrari, and starting to take greater care of it ,you will inevitably start asking yourself how you can also take greater care of your precious and invaluable home: Planet Earth. And by establishing practices that are not only conductive to your individual wellbeing but also to the greater good of all life on this planet, well that's how you'll start feeling like a real winner in life. And let me tell you, nothing and I truly mean nothing feels better than learning to live at that junction.

The beauty of this is that mother nature, in its infinite wisdom, has made it so that the healthiest way of living for us as individuals in most cases also has the greatest positive impact on the world as a whole so by improving in one area, you will inevitably also generate a positive impact on the other. I'll share more about this as we go on.

I know it can feel overwhelming and daunting to start thinking with such a wide perspective: some of the problems the planet is facing feel SO huge that one can easily feel discouraged to even start taking action. But humanity is nothing more than a very large group of individuals so transformation will indeed happen one person at a time. If everyone thinks that nothing can be done, that will be the case. But what if everyone started thinking that something SHOULD be done and started changing what they themselves do? Well let me tell you, that's precisely how we change the world!

All the changes and improvements we recommend come from this greater perspective: It's not merely about getting the best results in the fastest possible way. It is about achieving the most profound transformation at the root level, in the most sustainable way for yourself and all around you. So please bear this in mind as we move on and you'll see just how powerful the Shift really is.

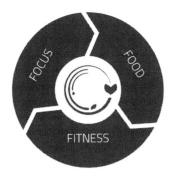

The Tripod Theory

I trust we're all familiar with what a tripod looks like: it's a structure with three legs that keep it upright. What happens to a tripod if even just one of the three legs is weaker than the other two? The whole structure is weak as a result of it and at risk of collapsing. It doesn't matter how strong one or two of the legs are, if one of them is weak, the whole structure is weak.

We've had the honor of working with over 500 professionals across 5 countries in our 20+ years of combined experience and the most valuable outcome has been that it has allowed us to identify the 3 pillars of wellbeing. These three fundamental areas are the three legs that sustain the structure of your optimal level of health and wellness.

One of the most common reasons why busy and time-pressed business owners struggle to achieve the results they would like to or, even more commonly, struggle to maintain these results, is that they're focusing on only one or two of the three pillars instead of all three. We see this happen time and time again: it's the reason why New Year resolutions don't work, it's the reason why we "fall off the wagon". It's one of the main reasons why most people who go through a "health kick" will, at some point or another, revert back to square one with a vengeance and find themselves even worse off than they started.

It's also the reason why individuals who may believe they've got a handle on their fitness and wellbeing, either because they train a lot or they eat very healthy, end up experiencing breakdowns or still feel like something is missing and they are unable to fulfill their overall potential.

As long as one of the three legs of the tripod is slightly weaker than the others, the structure as a whole is weaker. It doesn't matter how strong the other two legs are. The thing with us humans is that we love to do what we're good at more than what we're not so good at. So whenever we experience a loss of power, we will try our upmost to further improve what's already good to take it to the next level, rather than improving in an area we're completely lacking in. So if we're not feeling up to scratch in our fitness, we will try and do a bit more of what we know has helped in the past; we will try and improve a little further in something we already have a handle on. Essentially we will continue to strengthen the same one or two strong legs instead of working on the one leg that needs it most.

Another reason why this happens is because more often than not, we don't actually know what our weak areas are and one thing is for sure, you can't improve on something you're not even aware of. We can't spot our own blind spots (the clue's in the name!). Nobody can. I can't see my own blind spots and it doesn't matter how many people's health I've contributed to, how much knowledge I have, I will forever remain unable to spot my blind spots. That's why even the greatest athletes in the world have a coach: I mean does Roger Federer really need someone to tell him how to play tennis at this point? Surely he must know everything there is to know about tennis? Probably yes, but all the knowledge becomes irrelevant if he doesn't have someone from the outside looking in to give him a clear and objective perspective on the things he can't see by himself because they're in his blind spot. So if Roger wants to continue to stay at the top and get better and better, he needs to be constantly aware of his blind spots.

Identifying a blind spot within the tripod of wellbeing is like finding that little hole (or huge gash in some cases) in a tire that's causing it to deflate and lose its power. We often work with individuals that are doing many things right, puzzled why their greatest level of fitness and wellbeing is still escaping them. The reason will inevitably and invariably be found in the fact that they're not strengthening all three legs of the tripod equally, and there's an area they're not even aware of that is continuously being neglected.

Once you identify what this area is and start making incremental improvements to strengthen it, you'll be blown away by what you'll be able to accomplish. Not only will you progress faster than ever before, but you'll also be able to achieve results which are way greater than you ever thought possible. By strengthening all three legs of the tripod equally, simultaneously and systematically, you will be able to achieve far greater results in less time than if you go all-in and put all your efforts in developing only one or two of the legs.

So without further ado, let's go through these three fundamental pillars and why they're essential to you achieving your greatest level of health and wellbeing once and for all.

HERE'S A GAME CHANGING TIP:
Visit our website **www.wholeshiftwellness.com** and take 5 minutes to fill in our FREE and comprehensive scorecard questionnaire to help you identify the areas with most room for improvement across the three pillars of wellbeing.

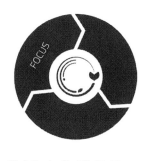

CHAPTER 3

Focus

Everything starts in the mind. You may have heard this saying before but have you ever actually stopped to contemplate what it truly means and how it affects your health and wellbeing?

We all know that our mindset is fundamental to our success but how many of us truly make a conscious and continuous effort to train our mind systematically? I did use the word "train" deliberately because we firmly believe that our mind needs as much (if not more) training and attention than our body.

If your mindset is not right, nothing else matters or will make a difference in the long run. An untrained mind will cause you to set unrealistic goals and then give up at the first hurdle. It will act on the self-sabotaging thoughts which are bound to show up along the way. It will make you revert back to what it's most used to because it's comfortable and predictable, rather than what has to happen to generate new results. It will find reasonable ways to justify doing the same thing over and over whilst expecting a new outcome (the very definition of insanity!)

This is the one pillar we regularly see being most neglected, which is unfortunate since it is the most important one and will make the greatest difference. Without a clear and strong strategy revolving around your Focus, you simply won't reach your goals and if you do, you'll find it very hard to maintain them in the long run.

Let me give you the most common example of how a lack of strategy around the Focus pillar may show up: the New Year resolution.

January 1st: "This is definitely the year things are going to change for me. I am full of confidence and determination, possibly more than ever before in my life. I just can't accept this any longer. I will lose 3 stone in 3 months come what may, and I will get back into those jeans from 1995 that I've been holding onto for dear life in the hope that the moment may come. This is the moment. Things are going to change NOW. I've hit rock bottom: I mean who eats THAT much Christmas pudding?! And for breakfast too?!? Disgusting and simply unacceptable. Not to mention the leftovers and mince pies. Unbelievable. All I want now is salad. I'm going to eat salad with no dressing for 3 solid months. Maybe a bit of soup here and there when I fancy something warm. That'll do it, surely. There's no way I should crave anything more than that after this shameful and excessive Christmas performance. I do really want it this year. It's different from all the other years when I tried this same thing but didn't last that long. This year I can sense it is different. Watch out world because nothing and I mean nothing can get in the way of losing 3 stone."

January 3rd: "See, I told you this year was different. It's been 3 solid days and I haven't touched anything other than salad and soup. Not even one bite. In fact, yesterday

I skipped a meal altogether. I may even try that juice cleanse the lady was talking about on the telly: maybe I should abstain from solid foods altogether for a month or so? This is the year I can do it because I'm telling you, I have a fire in my belly. It's truly different this time. I can't believe John had the audacity to bring mince pies in the office today. I mean, who does that?! I don't think I'll ever eat carbs at all ever again. I've already lost 6 pounds; I have a feeling I'll get to my goal in 2 months instead of 3. Check me out!! I'm on a roll!!"

January 6th: "I'm hungry. All day every day. Starving really but here's what's new this year: I actually don't mind it. I think I have developed the ability to just sustain hunger indefinitely. This must be how those celebrities do it. Sure it did take me every little bit of strength and willpower I have in me to resist that piece of bread the waiter brought over with the soup I ordered yesterday. But I did it! I resisted."

January 10th: "F***k this s**t. I can't believe this happened. I was doing so very good! F*****g John had to bring in that amazing lasagna for us all to share: I even told him what I was up to, with my new regimen! Selfish pig! "Just one piece won't spoil it for you" He said. What does he know? Of course it did. Since it was all ruined anyway, I went ahead and had one of those mince pies he keeps bringing in. It did taste amazing I must say. I ended up eating 3 of them and now ALL my efforts are out the window. All gone. What's the point in even kidding myself with this? I'm obviously broken. There must be a genetic predisposition to being slim that I simply don't have. I may as well go for drinks after work: that'll make me feel better about what a massive failure I am. They're going for curry afterwards, man I have been craving curry like mad this week. Oh well, beer and curry it is. I can always start again next week. Maybe I'll go straight into a juice cleanse next week because the thing is, if I don't eat solids at all, I may be able to resist all food. Yep, that's what I'll do. One last blow out this weekend then juice cleanse for a month from next week."

January 13th: "I know I said I was going to start a juice cleanse today but I have two birthdays and a work dinner this week. There's simply no way I can do it this week. We're even going to that amazing new restaurant everyone keeps talking about. I'll have to start next week."

I think you get where I'm going with the above. A poor mindset didn't cause the breakdown in the above example but it certainly is the root cause of the problem. We've all experienced something similar to some extent. It is the perfect example of how we set ourselves up for failure from the get-go by setting goals that are virtually impossible to maintain. We then try and stick to such goals with only will-power (a muscle which sooner or later will get tired and give up on us). We make up reasonable excuses which point the blame elsewhere when such silly plans inevitably fail. This vicious cycle ends up making us feel worse than when we started, so sooner or later, we give up and shamefully revert back to the old habit patterns.

The best way to spark long lasting change is to transform your mindset by going to the root level of what isn't working for you.

You've gotta dig deep. The deeper you dig the roots, the strong
this new seedling of wellbeing will be, the more it will be able to
face the elements, survive and grow against all odds. In our experience, we've been able to identify the 3 main actions you've got
to take to build a strong strategy around your Focus: these will act
like a Tripod within the Tripod making your structure of Focus
solid and strong.

Here they are.

Empty

Empty: the first fundamental action to take when building a strong mindset to support your goals is to Empty your mind of thoughts and belief systems which will sabotage your efforts. This is easier said than done as most of us feel powerless when it comes to controlling or even just directing our thoughts. We are trained to believe that thoughts are spontaneous and uncontrollable, they just happen to us and there isn't much we can do about that. Monkey Mind, they call it and for good reason. A mind that is not trained and directed will jump from one thought to the next uncontrollably like a monkey jumps from one branch to the next with no particular aim or direction. In reality, we have WAY more control over our mind than we tend to believe, but much like an untrained wild animal, if we never exert that control, it will do what it wants when it wants.

The first fundamental step in transforming your mindset therefore, is to realize and accept it is fully in your control and this can be quite confronting and overwhelming due to the simple fact that, generally speaking, we like to point the finger outside of ourselves. Thoughts like the following pop in our mind and it's so comforting and easy to believe them that we find very hard not to: "It is my mother's fault that I love sweets so much because she used to deprive me of them when I was little, so now I'm making up for that whenever I can" or "Overweight runs in the family, we're just all big like that, we all have a big appetite!" or even "it is John's fault that I broke my commitment to my New Year's resolution, if he hadn't bought that delicious food in the office, I wouldn't have broken all rules and gone wild". All these are example of self-sabotage due to blaming others and allowing our Monkey Mind to call the shots spontaneously, rather than directing it to do what we want it to do and what is most conducive to our happiness. Let me clarify, at this point, it is VERY difficult and virtually impossible to get rid of ALL non-conducive thoughts for good. There is an element of spontaneity to the thought process that is truly outside of our control HOWEVER we always are in control of what thoughts we believe and follow through on. We can always decide which thoughts to act upon and which thoughts we'll just witness and allow to wither away without them affecting us. If a non-conducive thought is merely witnessed without much reaction, slowly but surely the neuron-pathway that brings it to life will become weaker and weaker until one day that thought will stop coming up altogether. Empty therefore doesn't simply stand for emptying your mind of all thoughts or all negative thoughts, it is more the act of witnessing without reacting until such thoughts eventually lose all their potency and any control they may have over us. Now, let me tell you, this takes quite a bit of practice. There's nothing spontaneous about this and if you think that just by understanding how it works, you'll be able to change it, think again! Firstly, you've got to create a solid routine and strategy that allows you to identify what the main self-sabotaging thoughts are for you right now, pertaining to your current goals and aspirations. Then, you must practice witnessing them as and when they come up without reacting over and over and over again. Like, hundreds of times. That's why establishing a meditation routine of any kind is the single most empowering thing you can do to support you along the way.

The greatest misconception I often hear about meditation is that it's the "practice of not thinking" which sounds daunting and impossible because it is! Meditation is instead the practice of concentrating the mind on an object of our choice (sounds, mantra, breath or other) so that it stops wondering around aimlessly without any control and we can instead start regaining some control over it. And if an unwanted thought pops up whilst meditating, which will inevitably happen, we will bring the mind back to the object of focus time and time again without ever losing our cool. The moment you start practicing this daily, you'll find that you'll become more able to resist reacting to self-sabotaging thoughts and you'll gradually become more and more skilled at witnessing them before bringing the mind back to your chosen object.

Any little step you can take to introduce a mindfulness/meditation practice in your life will create profoundly positive results. It could be 5 minutes on one of the very popular apps that are around these days. Or it could simply be focusing on your breath for 5 minutes before you go to sleep. It may even be taking a walk with no distractions such as music, phones or other and just focusing closely on every little step you take. It could be Yoga.

The reason why those who practice it get so into it is because yoga allows you to work the body out whilst also detoxifying the mind. This could happen when one works out in any other way, however if you go to the gym, you'll find it is harder to concentrate the mind on one thing and one thing only as those environments tend to be set-up with plenty of distractions that give lots of branches to the Monkey Mind to hang from (loud music, loud people, noise from the equipment, TV screens etc). Whatever your chosen activity is, it truly doesn't matter but make sure that every single day you find a way to practice Emptying the mind by witnessing the thoughts as they come up without reacting to them.

Exercise: Look back at three instances when you broke your commitment to your wellness journey (whether it's not sticking to your eating plan or fitness/meditation routine). Identify the main thought which came up in each instance that justified you breaking your commitment to yourself: what did you say to yourself just before breaking your vow? Write these three thoughts down and notice if/how they may have come up at other times and in other circumstances too.

1. _____

2. _____

3. _____

Then write down three very strong answers to dispel them, so that if and when they come up next, you won't act on them.

1. _____

2. _____

3. _____

Concentrate

Concentrate: the act of emptying the mind of non-conducive thoughts (or at least learning not to act upon them) goes hand in hand with the act of Concentrating on your goals, aspirations and why. The more rehearsed you are on what you want to achieve and why, the easier it will be to stay on course until you reach your destination. This is totally worth spending some time on, so that you can really dig deep and find not only the superficial reasons that motivate you (lose some weight, fit into some item of clothing, run a certain distance in a certain time) but also and more importantly the deepest motivations.

I've seen this happen time and time again and can absolutely assure you that the greatest tools you have against self-sabotaging thoughts are your deepest reasons why you embarked on the journey in the first place. The deeper your why, the less likely you are to lose momentum and deviate from the course.

Most people we work with tell us that they have clear goals and motivations: that's why they're so puzzled that the ultimate result continues to escape them. Many of them are high achievers in other areas of life: they have a great career, great income, happy families and know that when they set their mind to something, they get it done and over achieve on what they set out to. Why is it then, that they can't lose a few pounds and keep it off for good? Why is something that on paper looks so simple, so hard for them to master? One of the main reason is that they actually tend to underestimate the real weight (pun intended) of what they're trying to achieve and most importantly, why they're trying to achieve it. They tend to be very clear on the full implications of not succeeding in the other areas of their lives which they mastered and that clarity is what keeps them motivated to excel and continue to get great results. When it comes to their health and wellbeing however, they only have a very superficial view of why it is important to them and have never spent enough time delving deep. This is precisely what keeps them stuck in a rut. They say it is important to them and are genuinely uncomfortable with the fact that they haven't been able to master this area of life but they continue to prioritize other activities because they're not fully present with how important their health and wellbeing REALLY is and the profound effects and repercussions of this lack.

Let me say now that I have absolutely nothing against goals such as losing weight or dress sizes, running marathons, wearing bikinis: I believe those can be powerful motivators and can be leveraged in useful ways. When the shit hits the fan however, as it inevitably will, it becomes very easy to make up excuses and believe the self-sabotaging thoughts if all you have against them is "I want to lose a dress size". You come up with things like: "I can eat less at the next meal to make up for it" or "I've already lost plenty, I can slow down a bit" or "I actually don't want to look too skinny, it doesn't suit me" or "just this one meal won't ruin it surely" or "I've walked a lot this week, I can skip the run"…and so on and so forth.

However, when you dig really deep into your motivations and find the ones that are most close to your heart, then trust me when I say that you'll become virtually unshakable in the face of doubt and temptation. One way to get to these deeply embedded motivation is to do an exercise I call "5 Whys". In fact, let's take a moment now for you to do this with me:

Exercise: Write down the top 3-5 wellness goals which in an ideal world, you'd love to achieve. There's no right or wrong answer here so simply note down the first 3-5 that come to mind.

1. _____

2. _____

3. _____

4. _____

5. _____

Now for each of them, ask yourself Why you want to achieve this goal at least 5 times. So for example, you may want to lose weight. Ask yourself Why you want to loose weight and see what comes up. Whatever thing comes up ask yourself why you want that. And so on and so forth. When you've done it at least 5 times and you're satisfied that you've identified your deepest reason, write that down next to your goal.

1. Goal _____

Deepest Reason _____

2. Goal _____

Deepest Reason _____

3. Goal _____

Deepest Reason _____

4. Goal _____

Deepest Reason _____

5. Goal _____

Deepest Reason _____

Trust me when I say that it is WAY easier to flag in the face of your Goal than it is to flag in the face of your deepest reason. They just have such a different weight! For example you may have realized that the deepest reason behind your goal of losing 1 stone is that you don't want to die prematurely like your father and not be able to meet your grandkids. How much easier is it to find an excuse against "losing weight" than "meeting your grandkids"? Yep, much easier.

The most fundamental reason why you have succeeded and smashed your goals in certain areas of your life but are still struggling with your health and wellbeing, is that you're not yet fully in touch with the real implications and deepest motivations. If you do nothing else, even if you don't finish the book, you should take the time to complete this exercise and actually write down your answers. Doing it "in your head" doesn't count one bit. You MUST put pen to paper. That's the only way that your brain is going to really register it and know that you mean business. Believe me when I say that simply completing this exercise will be such a catalyst for change that inevitably, your actions will reflect that even if only in a small way to begin with. Then if you REALLY mean business and are TRULY ready to reach your greatest level of health, wellbeing and life satisfaction, read on and see how you can best leverage on this exercise to transform your life in ways that you can't even imagine yet.

Reinforce

Reinforce: repetition is the mother of all skills. This could not be more true with regards to your health and wellness and it is the very thing that will make ALL the difference between you giving up three weeks into the process or staying with it until you've reached what you set out to do.

One of the greatest obstacles which gets in the way of busy and time-pressed professionals actually reaching their goals is, once they make up their mind on getting started, they want results to appear as fast as they can say "beach body". They've spent years, if not decades gradually losing track and building non-conducive habits, but they find it hard to spend a few weeks or months to improve and transform things for the better. This makes them easy bait to the myriad of short-term solutions available on the market; all the 21 days plans, 3 stones in 3 weeks, 7 days juice cleanses, potions, pills and other gimmicks of sorts which promise results that are nothing short of miraculous in the blink of an eye. Some of them even go into these things knowing they don't work. They say to themselves "I'll just do it to kick-start things and once I've lost a few pounds, I'll then continue just eating healthy". Unfortunately all results achieved in an unhealthy and unsustainable way will backfire with a vengeance sooner or later, and you'll find yourself back at square one with yet another failure under your belt to dent your confidence. It is WAY more effective and possibly less time consuming to accept and embrace the fact that it's going to take some time to reach your goals, but if you do so in a healthy and smart way, once you get there you will be there for good.

If it's taken you 10 years to get to where you are, it's unrealistic if not irresponsible to expect yourself to sort it all out in 10 days.

Even 10 weeks would be a bit of a stretch. What if it took you 10 months? Most people will gasp in horror at hearing such predictions: "a year?! It's going to take that long?! I have a wedding next month that I want to get to looking my best…"

Is a year really that long a time to undo 10 years (or more) worth of neglect? I really invite you to ponder this, as I know for a fact it is one of the greatest obstacles to real and long-lasting success. Many people have wasted years of their lives trying short-term fixes that didn't work time and time again, yet they're not prepared to commit a solid year to an approach that will genuinely bring forth profound transformation because it works at the root level of the issues. And even those who do decide to commit to a medium to long-term approach inevitably end up losing steam and motivation. This can always be traced back to a lack of Reinforcing their deepest whys and motivations.

It is powerful to go through the exercise above, addressing your deepest Whys but let me tell you what will truly take that exercise to the next level: Reinforcing those Whys every single day (or at least once a week) for the entire duration of whichever process you've committed to. Does this sound pedantic and repetitive? It is. But it works. In fact, it makes all the difference.

Anyone who has succeeded in any area of life will tell you that they had a way of keeping themselves engaged and motivated regularly and consistently. If you do the 5 WHYs exercise and write it all down as suggested, you'll get a new and exciting breeze of motivation that will start sparking new actions which will inevitably lead to new results. Those results however will take some time to show themselves to you in a tangible way.

For example, if you started saving up money or investing today, you would be starting to build momentum towards achieving financial freedom however, to begin with, the compound results of your efforts will seem pretty small and hardly tangible. The key is to not "stalk" the results but simply embrace the journey and trust the process in the full knowledge that you're definitely headed in the right direction, if you only stick with it for enough time. Now, let me tell you, the only way that you're going to stick with it for enough time to get to the final destination is if you remind yourself DAILY of why you embarked on the journey to begin with. You honestly can't do too much reinforcing, in fact most people don't do enough.

Just think about a loved one like your child or spouse: have you told them that you love them just once and then expected them to remember it for the rest of their lives? They know you love them right? What's the point of saying it over and over again? Surely they remember by now and would never question it.

Thankfully that's not how we approach it. Most of us express our love to those around us regularly. We constantly Reinforce the message to them and in fact, we do it even more when they're dealing with difficulties and need an extra reminder, right?

The same thing applies to reinforcing your commitment to your wellness journey. It needs to become such a deeply engrained habit that nothing will shake it and if things get rocky and you wobble along the way (it will happen!) you will go back to your deepest WHYs and reinforce them even more than usual in full knowledge that those are the times you need that most.

Here are some ideas of things you can do to Reinforce your motivation regularly:

1. Write your goals and motivations in bold on an A4 sheet and stick them up somewhere where you can see them daily (fridge, hallway mirror, bedside).
2. Take a picture of them, save it in your phone and set a reminder to look at the picture daily.
3. Save the picture as your screensaver on all electronic devices.
4. Talk about them openly with those you love so they can support you along the way.
5. Do a quick audio recording of them and keep it on your phone so you can listen to it at least once a week.
6. Create a vision board or collection of pictures and images that speak to your goals and 5 Whys.

Whatever you do, build a habit of doing it daily or weekly, and watch your motivation not only sustain itself but actually grow along the journey to your most fit, healthy and confident self.

A Note On Deprivation

Deprivation is a word that comes up time and time again in our sessions with clients. I wanted to take a minute to address it as we know it to be a massive obstacle on the road to success for many. What exactly is deprivation? It is nothing but an emotion. It arises when one feels like he or she is missing out on a pleasant and desired activity or item that one feels entitled to. The way it manifests itself in our mind is something along these lines:

> "Oh man, I wish I had a nice car like Mark over there. That's a seriously cool car, look how fly Mark looks riding around with the top down! I know I'm supposed to be saving up to buy a house right now but I'm so annoyed that I'm missing out on the joys and pleasures of riding a cool car! How is buying a nice house going to help with the ladies anyways? it's not like I can parade it around for them all to see? I'm telling you, I've got my priorities wrong. I'm gonna end up alone and miserable in my own home when I could have been happy and popular riding a fancy car around! And it's cheaper than a house too! I may just quit this saving and just splash the deposit I have accumulated so far on a fancy car like Mark has…"

So we have a plan that we've created with care and logic: saving money to buy a house. We know it's a sensible plan and we know why we're doing it: it's a long term plan but it will massively pay off once we see it through. We're delaying pleasure for a little while but in full knowledge that what we'll get as an outcome is totally worth it and way more than any short-term joy we may be having to miss out on at present. However, we can't help but compare and feel like what we're missing out on is worth more than what we're working towards. Hello Deprivation!

I'm sure you can see where I'm going but let's look at an example of how this applies to food.

So you had to attend your best friend's wedding and looking for an outfit was just the most dreadful experience. None of your old smart clothes fit properly any more. You just can't believe you've put on so much weight. It's ridiculous. You had to go around town trying more clothes that don't fit properly and settle for an outfit in a size that's painful to even think about. How could you let yourself go like this? It's ridiculous. You spent weeks being miserable about this and couldn't even fully enjoy the wedding in that horrible outfit you had to settle for. And now you've even started to get some weird pains that you never had before. You googled what it may be and what came up is actually quite worrying. You shouldn't have googled it because now you're feeling a little paranoid about life in general. You can't even sleep properly thinking about Google's diagnosis. This has to stop now. You're no nutritionist but it doesn't take a degree to know that eating cake or pastries every day is not gonna help the situation one bit. You're determined. Cakes are for special occasions, not every day meals. No. More. Cakes. At least not Monday to Friday. You know that's a smart starting point and have calculated that you would create a deficit of thousands of calories each week if you simply stopped the daily cakes and pastries. Surely that's bound to make a difference in a few months?! No brainer. It's happening. Cakes are out, new me is in!

Fast forward to the following day. A colleague is celebrating their birthday and they brought in a selection of cupcakes including your favorite: red velvet!

Oh my! Red Velvet is your absolute favorite! You haven't had one in ages and these look like very good ones: just the right amount of frosting. Look at that! But wait, what about the no cake on weekdays rule? Oh man! It sucks! Why can't you just be like David? He eats everything he wants and never puts weight on. Your life is so shit. This is your dad's fault, you inherited his slow metabolism and lack of fitness. You can't believe you have to miss out on your favorite cake. Look how everyone is enjoying this moment. It's not just about the cake, it's about the bonding experience with the team. You know they must all be thinking you're a looser for saying no to cake. They pretended to be supportive when you explained the no cake on weekdays rule but that's just because they pity you. You know in their mind they must be thinking you're a cake-avoiding-party-pooper. It sucks man. And it's probably not even going to make any difference. Cake or no cake, you're still plagued by your father's slow metabolism so the only way you could ever really lose weight is if you stop eating all the good stuff and what kind of a life is that?! A miserable one for sure. You may as well be miserable eating cake rather than be miserable and deprived of cake. Screw it. Pass me a red velvet!

And just like that, deprivation wins this battle. Now let me ask you a question: how long does it take to eat a red velvet cupcake? I'm guessing minutes. Personally, I could probably polish one off in two simple and swift bites, so for me it would actually only take seconds. So about 20-30 seconds of pleasure derived from the taste of red velvet in your mouth. If you eat one every day of the week, that's around 210 second of pleasure or 3.5 minutes.

Now let me ask you another question, how much does the discomfort of not being your most fit, healthy and confident self last? In the example above, you spent hours looking for outfits and feeling frustrated and worthless. Maybe as many as 6 hours. You couldn't fully enjoy your friend's wedding: so that's at least another 4-6 hours of feeling a bit low. Then you googled what your pains may be and are now feeling quite anxious every night before you go to bed, thinking about what Google told you it may be. In a week that could easily add up to another 7-10 hours of anxiety and worry. It's actually likely to be more but if you add it all up we're looking at anything between 17 and 22 hours of discomfort in one week.

The way you justify eating the cake is that you don't want to feel deprived. What deprives you more though? You can feel deprived from not experiencing the pleasure that comes from the taste of cake for around 3.5 minutes each week.

Or you could feel deprived by feeling bad emotionally and physically for as many as 22 hours in a week (generally more), which eating cake daily heavily contributes to.

Which deprivation has the greatest negative impact on your life? Which one takes most away from you? Which one weights more heavily on your body, mind and soul? I know my answer, but what's yours?

Many come to me telling me they are worried about changing their eating because they don't want to stop "enjoying life" or "having all the fun" or "miss out on the pleasures of living":

how much fun, joy and pleasure is there in going around feeling unfit, unhealthy, and lacking confidence, and in many cases, even worrying that chronic disease is just around the corner?

Deprivation is a trick of the mind. But that's great because it means that you can use it to your advantage! Instead of focusing on all that you're missing out from not eating cake (i.e. minutes of pleasure), shift the focus constantly onto all that eating cake daily deprives you of. Or even better, shift the focus onto all that eating healthy foods will give you: the joy of feeling fit, healthy and confident every hour of every day. The pleasure of going shopping and buying whatever outfit you want because most things look good on you. The joy of sleeping soundly at night in full confidence that you're doing your best to take the best possible care of your wellbeing. The pleasure of feeling confident in your own skin and exuding positive energy to everyone around.

Exercise: What are your 3 most unhealthy habits and what do they deprive you of?

1. Habit _____

Deprivation _____

2. Habit _____

Deprivation _____

3. Habit _____

Deprivation _____

Fun Fact

Did you know that the pleasure you get from eating something delicious gradually decreases as you keep eating it? This is true on a neurological level and has been scientifically proven. The first bite is the one that will spark the most pleasure by stimulating the greatest neurological response, especially with food that contains highly stimulating substances such as refined sugars and lots of fat. All subsequent bites will gradually generate less and less positive response as the body gets gradually used to the substance. Because we get so much pleasure from the first bite, we keep eating more and more in an effort to re-create it, when in fact we're going further and further away from it. Like with drugs and any other stimulants, the body gets used to them so one needs to continuously increase the quantity in order to spark the original response. This concept is beautifully explained at length in one of my favorite books on health and nutrition: The Pleasure Trap by Dr. Lisle. Highly recommended.

****

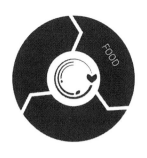

CHAPTER 4

Food

Here's something we always say to our clients to emphasize the importance of nutrition: you can't outrun a bad diet, no matter how fast you go. I truly believe that some of the most unlucky people out there are those who can get away with eating junk all day long without ever putting on weight. Yes, you read that right: I think an ultra-fast metabolism that doesn't allow for weight gain is actually a curse rather than a blessing. And a very dangerous one at that.

Here's why: if you could eat all the junk in the world without ever putting on weight, what do you think you would end up doing? Most of us would end up eating all the junk in the world for as long as we possibly could, because let's face it: if it doesn't affect our external appearance, surely it doesn't matter so much, right? Wrong. Dangerously wrong.

The negative impacts of bad eating habits go WAY deeper than your physical appearance. In fact that may just be the least important implication, but unfortunately, it's the one we seem to care about the most these days. The food you eat is the fuel for the most precious machine you will ever own in this life: your body.

Now I've said this before, if you owned a Ferrari (maybe you do, lucky you!), would you fuel it with the cheapest, lowest grade fuel you can get your hands on or would you go out of your way to find the best quality fuel there is on the market? This applies even more to your body.

Luckily nature has designed things so that actually, the best fuel for your body is some of the most inexpensive out there.

Unfortunately, the world we live in has low grade food-like products more readily available that the food we should be eating, so these days, it does take some effort to feed your body the fuel it needs and deserves, but trust me when I say, the effort is SO worth the outcome.

Even if you work out a lot and burn a lot of calories or if you're one of those lucky few who can get away with eating anything, I cannot emphasize enough the importance of learning to eat and enjoy healthy food. The negative effects of bad nutrition are profound and when you don't have vanity as an incentive, you're likely to push it to the point where you will suffer from chronic disease later on in life. I firmly believe that nobody gets away with a poor diet. Even those who look great will never be able to achieve their greatest level of health, fitness and mind-body confidence until they feed their Ferrari with the highest quality fuel they can get their hands on at all times.

Having said all that, I must also add that Food is always the most contentious subject and one of the most sensitive topics we unpack with our clients. Even those who completely realize and appreciate the importance of improving their nutrition, often have to overcome many stumbling blocks and hurdles in order to get there.

This is because our relationship with food goes far beyond what it should: fueling our bodies for survival. It is in fact an area of deeply embedded emotions and habits that often have deep roots in our past.

I haven't met many people who simply "eat to live"; most of us, to some degree or another, "live to eat". That's why the Food pillar and the Focus pillar MUST be worked on and developed closely: you'll find that, more often than not, what you perceive to be a challenge revolving around Food is, in fact, one that more predominantly revolves around Focus. Everything starts in the mind and the food choices we make every day are a direct result of our belief systems.

Many come to us believing that if they could simply receive a detailed food plan that they can follow scrupulously for the duration of the program, they wouldn't have to make decisions or think about food and that would resolve all their problems. I won't lie to you, I used to believe that myself. Whenever I used to put some weight on (and many times it was A LOT of weight on), I used to fool myself that all I needed was a strict but clear step-by-step eating plan that I could just follow for some months fueled by lots of willpower, and all my problems (and extra pounds) would go away.

But just stop and think for a moment: if this approach really worked, in fact, if diets worked, would we ever need to do more than one in our life? If all we need is a strict set of rules to follow with willpower for a period of time, why is it then that even some of the smartest people I've ever met struggle sticking to a diet and end up either giving up or putting all the weight back on (and more) as soon as said diet is over? That's because the approach is faulty at the root level. DIETS. DON'T. WORK. They never have and never will.

The very concept is faulty: enduring a restrictive plan for a short period just for the sake of weight loss and then hoping to maintain the weight loss after the plan is over doesn't work. And those who actually go into such restrictive plans with the illusion that they will stick with them for the rest of their lives, will struggle just as much. That's because willpower should be viewed as a muscle and if you try to "muscle" your way to permanent transformation, you'll have a challenging time because sooner or later that muscle will get fatigued and give up on you.

I've been vegan since 2014 now and most of the week, I eat the "Whole Food Plant Based" way (that's unprocessed plant foods with no added sugar, salt or oil). I can assure you it takes zero willpower to eat the way I do. Zero. My commitment to the way I eat doesn't come from me "doing what I have to do"; It comes from me "doing what I want to do". It's a small detail that makes ALL the difference.

For example, think about a past boyfriend or girlfriend you used to be obsessed about but you've now long since moved on. Do you go around life having to use tons of willower not to call him/her up every day? Of course not. You don't even think about picking up the phone because you've outgrown them. There's no temptation, therefore there's no need for willpower.

The same applies to eating: I don't crave the processed, junky food I used to eat, ever. Sure once a week we'll go to a restaurant and I'll eat whatever vegan option I feel like, even if it's more processed and elaborate than my usual weekly choices but that's pretty much as far as it goes for me now. And no, I'm not special or different from anyone else.

Our clients go through exactly the same transformation. We work with them in such a way that healthier food simply becomes the new norm, not because they have to but because they want to. It's what they do. In fact, it becomes who they are. They become the kind of person who eats healthy most of the time and they're not tempted to do otherwise because they're too present with the pros and cons of their choice. It becomes a matter of Free Will instead of Willpower. They choose to eat well because they want to, so it's virtually impossible to sway them in another direction most of the time.

This process takes time of course, especially if you choose to go about it on your own; the sad truths is that you'll be more likely to give up before you experience the amazing results of this shift in consciousness that could fuel your success in the long run. Once you nail this however, even if it takes several attempts, life will never be the same again; you'll be able to achieve things that once felt imaginable. Way greater than you could ever imagine.

Read on for the top 3 areas to address if you want to improve your nutrition and, more importantly, the 5 proven steps to do so in a way that will transform your approach once and for all.

More Water

Sounds obvious right? However most people we work with grossly underestimate how much water they need to function optimally through the day and often assume that all liquids ingested count towards their daily consumption. Sadly, alcohol and coffee have quite the opposite effect on our body to hydrating it, and many other soft drinks contain so much sugar, artificial sweeteners and other harmful additives, that the positive effects of the water content are cancelled out by the negative effects of all the other "ingredients".

We are 60% water so going through life in a state of constant de-hydration can have a very profound negative impact on your productivity, vitality, energy levels and general health.

Many believe that because they don't sweat profusely or work out, they don't need to replenish water as much but the truth is that on any average day, you will lose at least 1.8 liters of water through perspiration and that is before you even hit the gym.

Your brain and heart are the two organs that contain the most water: they are in fact 73% water; so even a slight level of de-hydration (as little as 2%) can severely impair their functioning.

Without enough water, the organs will not get enough oxygen and nutrients to function optimally which, in the brain's case can lead to: headaches, dips in energy, lack of focus and memory loss. When the brain is dehydrated, it literally shrinks in size which causes it to pull away from the skull, this will result in the painful feeling we know as a headache.

Next time you feel one arising, instead of reaching for a painkiller, why not down a pint of filtered water or brew yourself a large mug of herbal tea (the only hot drink that counts towards your daily water intake)? See what happens.

This tip also applies to next time you feel lethargic and in need of an energy boost. We tend to reach for a treat or the second (or 5th) cup of coffee but those are generally short lived solutions with negative side effects, whereas you truly have nothing to lose by downing a large glass of water before you take further action.

Water is also fundamental for flushing toxins out of your body and aiding good digestion and elimination, which are also a great way to get rid of toxins; guess how you'll feel when you have less toxins stagnating in your blood stream and organs? that's right, freaking awesome! That's why a super sweaty workout, as hard as it may be, also feels so amazing: because by increasing the amount of water you "lose" you're also increasing the amount of toxins you lose. You will also feel more thirsty, which will lead to drinking more water, and in turn, yet more stale toxins being flushed out of the system. Win, Win, Win.

Another organ that will benefit profoundly from an increase in water consumption is actually the largest organ in the body: your skin. It is a whopping 64% water but because it is the most superficial organ, water will reach all other organs before it reaches your skin, making it more prone to suffer from dehydration. A lack of proper hydration will make your skin tight, flaky and more prone to wrinkles. Oh yes, I did say that, so if you're looking for a more radiant and younger looking complexion, you better drink up!

Lastly, by drinking more water you will prevent cravings and overeating: We often misinterpret the body's signals and what we believe to be hunger may in fact be thirst. It is very helpful to drink a large glass of water before eating. This will replenish any fluids that may be missing and contributing to a sense of lack/craving. Drinking water before a meal will also allow you to not be completely starving when you reach for the food, which can lead to eating more than you need. It will also aid digestion if you drink before instead of immediately after a meal, preventing bloating and dilution of your digestive enzymes.

5 Tips to increase your daily water intake:

1. Drink a large glass of water (ideally warm and maybe even with a few drops of lemon juice) as soon as you get up in the morning every day: start with a 350ml glass and gradually move up to 500ml. If you're an over achiever like myself, you can even work on getting through a whole liter of water first thing so that no matter what happens through the day, you know you're half way through your RDA before you've done anything else.

2. If you're not used to the taste of plain water or want to spice it up, add some fresh fruit of your choice. I love lemon juice but you can get as creative as you like. Slices of orange, cucumber, mint. The sky is the limit and whatever works to incentivize you.

3. Swap some of your coffees or black teas for herbal teas. Those are really the only hot drinks that count toward your daily water consumption since they have no counterproductive additives such as sugar, artificial sweeteners and other so you can drink as much as you like and you'll get all the same benefits as plain water.

4. Carry a refillable bottle with you at all times. That's one sure way that you're never going to be caught unprepared and it will also allow you to track your intake throughout the day, and notice if you've been staying on top of it of if you need to rev up the drinking a bit.

5. When you go out for a well-deserved Friday night pint (or two), always have a glass of water in between each alcoholic drink. This sounds like a painful and fun-spoiling habit but how much fun is it to wake up the next morning feeling terrible? How about trying a subtle compromise that will allow you to have fun with your mates whilst also not suffering for hours as a result of said fun? Sounds like a no brainer to me.

Learn to love your sweat and get the most out of it (pun intended!). Here are some reasons why:

1. Embrace it as a beautifying process but most importantly, learn to let it flow, quite literally! Some of the most harmful things you can do is using those anti/perspiration deodorants that lock the sweat inside your body. Think of it this way, you're literally locking in toxins! The body is trying to get rid of something bad and harmful via its largest organ (the skin) and you're putting on it a thick layer of harmful chemicals that prevent it doing its job! Not good!

2. Stop blasting the air-conditioning on max when working out. You're missing out from the greatest added benefit of the work-out: sweating out toxins and fat bi-products. Not to mention, a workout in warm conditions will burn WAY more calories than a workout performed in a cool

environment. This is because the body has to work harder to maintain its core temperature, resulting in more calories and fat burned. Your body releases heat through sweat, which comes from blood pumped to your skin. The hotter your body gets, the more blood your heart needs to pump to expel that heat.

3. Another very common mistakes we witness time and time again, especially when teaching Bikram yoga in 40' degrees heat, is that students will come in with a little towel and constantly reach for it to dry the sweat off their face and body. How many times do you think you would have to dry your sweat when practicing challenging hatha yoga poses in 40' heath for 60-90 minutes? That's right, hundreds! This is not only a waste of energy (your sweat is there to cool you down, the more you wipe it, the more you'll sweat) but also, most importantly, counterproductive from the perspective of detoxification because you're constantly pushing back in all the toxins that are trying to make their way out of your body.

More Plants

2014 was the year of BIG wins for me. On the 20th of June 2014 I married my soulmate, which was beyond surprising, given that just over a year prior I didn't even know him nor did I believe in soulmates. Then, on the 15th of August 2014, I stopped eating all animal products and haven't looked back since, which was another a huge surprise not only because It came "out of nowhere" but also because I was pretty certain it wasn't going to work for me.

The reason behind my decision to "try the plant-based thing" actually has nothing to do with food so I will leave it alone for now and may tackle it in my next book.

What I will say is that before I made the shift, I honestly felt I had achieved the greatest level of success and balance I could with my eating and I thought there was no way to improve things further. I thought that the only way I could continue to improve my level of physical and mental fitness was through exercise and medita-tion. So when the thought first arose to "try the plant-based thing", I pushed back. For weeks. Why would I mess around with habits that I was generally very happy with and that took me years to accomplish? Plus, going Vegan means having to eat Carbs and there was no way I was going to go down that road because for sure, that would have meant gaining weight. I may not have been looking to lose more weight but I also sure wasn't looking to put weight back on!

But the thought continued to come up with a vengeance so at some point my husband said: "Let's just try it and If it doesn't work, we can always go back. There's no harm in trying it for a while so you can get it out of your system. I'll do it with you". And try we did. We went all in actually, cleared the house of anything we decided to stop eating for a while and delved deep into plant based eating "for a month". Then something magical and completely unexpected happened that I genuinely never saw coming. At age 31 and after years of trials, tribulations, trying every diet under the sun, trying no diet at all and anything in between, I started unlocking the absolute greatest level of health, fitness, wellbeing and mind-body satisfaction I have ever been able to achieve in my entire life. I got in better shape than I was in my teens and twenties, no joke.

I resolved chronic issues I had been dealing with which I had gotten so used to, I didn't even perceive them as problems any longer (digestive difficulties, constipation, seasonal infections, horrible PMS, mood swings, cravings, energy dips, bloating, the list goes on). The weight started dropping off me without me even trying in fact, I was eating more food than before and still losing weight. My skin got clearer than ever before. My hair got shinier than ever before. Most importantly, my Soul got lighter than ever before. I can truly say, I've never looked back since and, together with yoga and meditation, plant based eating is one of the greatest sources of health, vitality and joy in my entire life. Hands down.

Now if you think that I'm saying all this because I want everyone to go fully plant based right now, you're wrong! One very important thing I learned from our own transition is that going all out, cold turkey the way we did can be counter-productive. It can be so hard, in fact, that it often leads to demotivation and overwhelm, which will in turn eventually lead to you giving up altogether, thinking it's not for you.

You don't have to go fully plant based to start experiencing amazing results and profound transformation. All you've got to do is: Eat More Plants! One of our shifters lost 6 kgs in 6 months by introducing some intermittent fasting into his weekly routine and eating WAY more plants than ever before. We educated him into realizing that he didn't need to "top-up" all his meals with animal protein in order to be healthy (adding a can of tuna on the quinoa salad, having eggs for breakfast at every possible occasion, having meat or chicken at every meal) so he started enjoying many fully plant based meals and snacks every week in the full knowledge that he wasn't "missing out" on anything necessary to his body. The weight fell off and his confidence and vitality soared, which was so inspiring to witness.

I won't go into technical detail around nutritional science as that would take an entire book on its own.

This is not because I don't know a lot more about nutrition than many GPs and doctors out there. Unfortunately, most doctors are not taught anything about nutrition over their many years of studying human physiology (they will confirm this themselves). Getting nutrition tips from your GP sadly may be just as valuable as asking the owner of your local corner store what he recommends you eat for breakfast.

If you want to learn technical information from some of the most prominent authorities on the topic, I highly recommend three incredible books that have profoundly impacted my life for the better in ways that were unimaginable and have transformed the views and wellbeing of all our shifters:

1. *The China Study*, by Dr. T. Colin Campbell
2. *Proteinaholic*, by Dr. Garth Davis
3. *How Not To Die*, by G. Stone and Dr M. Greger

The other reason why I'm not going to delve too deep into technicalities, is because I can assure you, hands down, that you don't need to know all the finer details in order to unlock your greatest level of health, fitness and wellbeing. I often find, in fact, that excessive focus on small details and technical information can be highly counterproductive. Sure, it makes us professionals sound quite clever to talk about Macros and Micros, essential amino-acids, water soluble or fat soluble vitamins etc. but trust me when I say that the reasons why you're overweight and unfit have very little to do with a lack of such knowledge. You don't need a degree to know that cleaning your plate as well as your kids' plate at every meal may not be the way forward. Nor do you need a degree to know that pints, cheese burgers and fries are not gonna get you there. You also don't need to know much about Macros to realize that the cake counter is not where you'll find a suitable snack on a week day. Or that pastry and muffins do not constitute a "healthy and nutritious breakfast".

By starting to address the lowest-hanging fruits, the very obvious stuff, the habits that you already know are not conducive to your goals, you will achieve greater results than you can even imagine and that has 0% to do with acquiring more knowledge on nutrition and 100% on shifting your Focus (as mentioned above). But we are so overwhelmed and confused by the myriad of information out there, most of which is actually conflicting, that we end up not knowing where to start from and never making any changes at all.

For now, all I want to emphasize on the subject are the following points:

1. Although you do need protein to live, you don't need as much as they would have you think.

2. Plants have protein. Plenty of it. You actually don't need to eat animal products in order to consume enough protein

3. Eating more protein doesn't help weight loss (it often does the opposite, as thoroughly explained by Dr. Davis in his book Proteinaholic)

4. The key to transforming your eating is to stop viewing food as their individual nutrient component (protein, carbs, fat) and start viewing it at a whole food item. This will help you make healthier choices right away. For example the reason why doughnuts and cakes are not an ideal snack and should not be eaten daily is NOT because they are (or have) Carbs. Bananas also have carbs but it doesn't take a scientist to figure out that bananas are a healthier daily snack than cakes and doughnuts.

5. 80-90% of what you perceive to be "Food" problems in your life, are actually "Focus" problems. You won't solve your FOCUS problems by acquiring more nutrition knowledge. You'll solve them by hiring a coach that can spot them when they're in your blind-spot and keep you accountable when you face the inevitable ups and downs you'll encounter along the way to success.

Want to learn more on this topic? check out my e-book called "6 Steps to Eat More Plants Without Feeling Deprived", available on **http://www.wholeshiftwellness.com**

More Natural

Natural food is the best food. It is as important to switch towards less processed food items as it is to eat more plants. The two things should go hand in hand and just doing a lot of one of them, may not be enough to achieve incredible results and profound transformation.

Are you reading this and struggling to clearly identify in your mind what "natural food" really is? Well I'll make this really simple for you: natural food doesn't have ingredients. Natural food IS ingredients. Apples, Bananas, Nuts, Rice, Potatoes, Beans or even spices such as paprika, chili, cinnamon, pepper, ginger : these are all as natural as they get. They are what they are. They don't require further explaining, nor do they require a degree in biology or biochemistry to know what they are. Dishes and meals that are made of a combination of natural foods (including spices) are always the best choices you can make.

If a food item has a long label containing very many ingredients, some of which sound like they could just as well be listed on your toothpaste or dishwasher tablet, it is safe to say it is NOT natural.

The more natural your food, the healthier you'll be. Of course, natural foods are NOT free of calories so it is still very possible to be overweight if you eat way more than you need, and this is especially true if you eat a lot of animal products for the simple fact that those are way more calorie-dense than plants. But if you've got to choose between a chemically sweetened, zero calorie soda and a freshly pressed organic juice that contains calories, I would pretty much ALWAYS recommend the natural juice. The goal, in my mind, is not to lose weight at all costs. The goal is to achieve your greatest level of health, fitness, wellbeing and life satisfaction and I can assure you, zero calorie processed food is not the route to such destination.

This is for two main reasons: the first one is that many of the chemical additives used in food production have actually been proven to be detrimental to human health. Why are they allowed to be used, you may ask? Great question and one that may also require a book to itself but the short answer is that highly profitable and powerful food manufacturers have found creative ways to manipulate a system they virtually own, in order to do what's most convenient to them. The chemical additives that have not yet been proven harmful have simply not been researched enough, so they may very well be, we just don't know yet. Now I'm not saying that you will get sick immediately if you eat a processed food item but I would discouraged anyone from routinely consuming them on a daily or even weekly basis.

The second reason is that, in order to function optimally, your body doesn't simply need a certain amount of calories, it actually also needs a minimum amount of nutrients. One of the most common reasons for cravings is that many individuals out there simply don't reach this minimum nutrient intake every day because they rely on highly processed foods, therefore they may be getting enough calories; in fact many of them get WAY more calories than they need, but since they're not getting enough nutrients, the body is constantly "looking and asking for more". Hence the constant craving.

Have you ever noticed how, after eating a very processed fast food meal, you literally feel like you could have it all over again? You may have just consumed 1,000 to 2,500 calories depending on what you ate exactly, but you feel like you've barely eaten at all.

You're barely satisfied and in fact are craving way more: for sure you can squeeze in a chocolate milk shake after the double cheese burger and large fries with soda!

Processed "food" is designed to make you want more, endlessly. It is created in laboratories, not kitchens, by scientists, not cooks. The cooks may execute it but the recipe is carefully designed to stimulate the dopamine centers in your body so that such "food" generates chemical reactions that are virtually impossible to resist and control. Once you start eating certain "foods" it is very hard to stop (some of them are even advertised as such) and you will not feel fully satisfied until you reach the point of feeling sick and disgusted.

On top of all this, processed "food" does not contain many nutrients. It contains plenty of calories, way more than you'll ever need. It may even contain enough macro nutrients (carbs, protein, fats. Definitely plenty of fats) but it never contains enough micro nutrients, therefore after a processed meal, your body will still be starving for the essential stuff it needs to function optimally and therefore it will continue to ask for it.

The general rule of thumb is this: the less processed food you eat, the better. This may not be the only solution to achieve your greatest results yet, but it certainly will take you very many steps forward.

Here's a quick, 3 steps approach to decrease your consumption of processed food.

1. Identify the top 3 offenders in your routine at present: keep a food journal for one week to log every single item of food you consume and read all labels. Sounds tedious but you can only improve what you're aware of and soon enough you'll build the awareness required to not have to do all this.

2. Substitute: research marginally less processed alternatives to your current top 3 offenders. Huge tip: don't get too extreme here. It is unrealistic for you to transition from Pringles to carrot sticks without hating every moment of it and wanting to go back to the highly stimulating and addictive taste of Pringles. It is WAY smarter to go from Pringles, to a more natural brand of crisps with no chemical additives and flavors such as the Eat Natural snacks or even Pop Chips or Walkers oven baked. Your taste buds may still rebel to begin with as they're used to much greater stimuli but they will gradually adapt.

3. Repeat: once the transition has become second nature and an effortless routine, repeat the process with the next top 3 offenders OR go back to the crisps and make another marginal improvement such as switching to pretzels or trail mix etc.

The tendency is to get restless and want to go from one hundred to zero. This leads to massive difficulties which leads to most people giving up before they've even had a chance to experience the great results of their improved habits. In wellness, much like in life, slow and steady wins the race.

A quick note on natural animal products. While it's true that natural foods are the best foods, consuming a lot of animal products, as natural as they may be, will still prevent you from reaching your greatest level of health, fitness and wellbeing. Organic, grass-fed beef and free-range chicken are better than a McDonald's burger and KFC bucket but eating steak every day is not the route to success. Many of our clients come to us puzzled as to what it is they're doing wrong: "we eat very well" they say. "Only organic. The best quality products we can get our hands on. No fast food. No processed food". Why is it then that they don't feel healthy? Why can't they lose weight?

"It's the carbs" they confess to me. "I just can't resist the bread basket". Then we look at their weekly food logs to discover that they're eating eggs and bacon for breakfast every day, steaks for lunch, salmon fillets for dinner and cheese for dessert. Yet, in their mind, the problem is the four pieces of bread they ate at the restaurant on Friday. The moment they switch from eggs to oats, steaks to beans and salmon to potatoes, the weight literally falls off them. They eat as much if not more than they did before, they feel full and satisfied yet they lose more weight than they've ever lost before and feel much better inside and out. Natural is good. Natural plants are best.

A quick note on processed vegan food: these days, we are definitely spoiled for choices when it comes to plant based food however it is important to remember that switching from animal products to highly processed vegan junk food will only marginally improve your health and wellbeing and may not be conducive to weight loss. The overall aim should still be to shift towards natural foods as much as possible. Vegan cheeses, meats and snacks can make for great transitional foods, especially in the early stages of shifting towards more plant based meals. When our taste buds are so used to the "strong" flavors of meat and cheese, it can be easier to go for a vegan processed option and that's completely fine. But it shouldn't be the ultimate goal. The ultimate goal remains to learn to love food that is consumed for the most part as found in nature (fruit, vegetables, root vegetables, legumes, grains, spices, herbs and also wholegrain flour products such as bread and pasta which are only minimally processed) because that is where you'll get the most amount of nutrition for the least amount of calories.

Dismantling Food Myths

These days we don't lack information. In fact we often have the opposite problem: an overload of information, some of which conflicting, which ends up confusing us and will inevitably lead to no improvements at all because a confused mind does nothing.

Although there are many different ways to improve your eating and get results, we are huge fans of wholistic improvements. We do not promote weight loss at all costs. Instead, we believe in mastering the most sustainable approach not only for you (so that you can create permanent transformation instead of temporary change) but also for the world and everyone around you. In our experience, this long term, wholistic approach is precisely what will unlock your greatest level of health, wellbeing and overall life satisfaction.

With all that said, let's unpack what I believe to be some of the most harmful misconceptions revolving around nutrition so that you can move on in an empowered way and can start making better choices right away. Please bear with me as I'm fully aware that some of what I'll say will massively challenge what's commonly believed to be true and may therefore take some time to digest.

I myself had to initially take many huge leaps of faith in accepting some of these truths. I wrestled in my own mind, not to mention in my daily exchanges with friends and family, with all the food myths that discourage plant based eating.

But nothing is more powerful than experiential knowledge in my opinion, as it is grounded in reality rather than just theory. What truly convinced me without any reasonable doubt of the legitimacy of these uncomfortable truths have been, above all else, the results that I have achieved in my own life, on my own skin as well as the incredible results achieved by our clients through the years.

So without further ado, let's delve into them:

1. **Carbs make you fat.** I was SURE I was going to gain weight from all the carbs I would have to eat on a plant based diet. In fact, I had made peace with the fact. So strong was the messages my body was sending me against meat consumption that I had accepted weight gain as a possible side effect of my shift. Needless to say, not only did I NOT put on weight, I actually lost more and more effortlessly than ever before in my life. The truth is, not all carbs are created equal. For sure, if you eat a lot of refined products such as white pasta, white bread and cakes (which actually have way more fat in them than carbs) you will hinder your weight loss effort and actually run the risk of not getting enough essential nutrients. However if you focus your efforts on eating plenty, and I mean PLENTY, of whole foods and wholegrains, you will simply fuel the body, especially your brain, with its primary source of energy (glucose) and eat a naturally low fat diet. I have never eaten so much (my portion sizes have more than doubled since going plant based) and weighed so little in my entire life. No joke. If you want to read more on this subject, I highly recommend a book called "The low carb fraud" by Dr McDougall. But the only way you will ever really be convinced is by trying this out for yourself: that's the only way my clients finally shift their thinking. Once you realize you DON'T have to be hungry and deprived to be in great shape, nobody else will be able to change your mind ever again.

2. **You can't get enough protein on a plant based diet.**
The protein question comes up time and time and time again. If I had a penny for every time someone asks "where do you get your protein from?" I would be retired and living on a desert island (and finally wouldn't have to hear the question ever again!). The truth is, plants have protein, and plenty of it. Or at least plenty to fulfill our human needs. I can't speak for lions and tigers. This huge misconception that pollutes our mind goes back hundreds of years and is often used as a marketing ploy by the food and supplement industry (they've gone as far as inventing protein enhanced water now!). Protein deficiency is virtually impossible if enough calories are consumed and is even harder if consuming plenty of nutrient rich foods such as fruits, vegetables, legumes and starches. I have personally logged my food intake for weeks at a time into Cronometer (the best food logging app out there) and have NEVER had a day when I hadn't consumed MORE than enough of the essential amino acids our body needs to build protein. The myth of "perfect protein" confuses the public: we are led to believe that animal protein is better because it is more similar in composition to our own body but actually, according to the World Health Organization (which has now officially classified processed and red meat as a class A carcinogenic) animal protein is anything BUT perfect. Dr. Garth Davis expands on this huge misconception in his INCREDIBLE book "Proteinaholic", which is one of the most interesting books you will ever read on nutrition (second only to "The China Study" by T. Colin Campbell). So the moral of the story is, don't worry about protein; simply focus on getting enough calories from a wide variety of nutrient-dense plant food and you will

be just fine. Actually, you'll be better than fine: you will thrive!

3. **We need milk for calcium.** Milk contains calcium, that's an indisputable truth. However there is compelling scientific evidence showing that consumption of dairy products is strongly associated with many diseases (constipation, skin problems, asthma, digestive problems and even cancer) making it FAR from the ideal source of calcium. It is no surprise that millions of people out there struggle to digest milk and complain of milk related allergies. We're simply NOT meant to be consuming milk from another mammal and especially not after weaning. Milk is also often contaminated with bacteria, hormones and antibiotics (routinely fed to cows to maximize mass-production). Not to mention the horrible conditions milking cows have to sustain for the entirety of their lives. Calcium is abundant in many plant based foods such as tofu, molasses, leafy greens and seeds: by getting it from plants, you avoid all the side effects of dairy consumption and will probably also lose a few pounds from the decrease in fat and hormones consumption. Dr. Campbell expands in depth on the negative effects of dairy consumption in his incredible book "The China Study", delving into the MOST comprehensive study of nutrition ever compiled in the history of humanity. This is a read I highly recommend to ALL my clients as it clearly and scientifically expands on why we should all ditch the dairy once and for all. Don't listen to me – just read his book. His credentials as a PHD and lab scientist with over 40 years of experience in nutrition studies are WAY more substantial than mine will ever be!

4. **We need fish for Omega 3 fatty acids.** Guess where fish get their omega 3 from? That's right, plants! So why not cut out the middle-man and avoid exposure to all the unhealthy substances found in fish? Some of these are, for example: saturated fat, cholesterol and heavy metals such as mercury. The idea that fish is a "healthy" choice probably comes from the belief that populations who eat fish are generally healthier than those consuming a meat rich diet. This may in fact be true but it's not the fish consumption that makes them healthier, so much as the decreased consumption of meat! Sure your diet will improve if you go from eating cheese burgers and fries to eating steamed fish and vegetables. You will also improve your health if you go from smoking crack to smoking cigarettes or from smoking a pack a day to smoking one; however that doesn't mean that smoking one cigarette a day is actually good for you. If you want to achieve optimal health and minimize as much as possible any exposure to toxic substances, you really need to avoid ALL animal products including fish and get your Omega 3 from the much healthier and abundant plant based sources out there such as flaxseed, chia seeds, walnuts and edamame and algae.

Eat Like An Empire Builder

In his book "Entrepreneur Revolution" our brilliant mentor and dear friend Daniel Priestley (co-founder of Dent Global, a company which specializes in helping businesses stand out and scale up whilst resolving the world's most meaningful problems) talks extensively about how to shift your mindset into "entrepreneurial" gear. He explains how we have three fundamental parts of the brain that have evolved at different stages in the evolution of mankind to serve a different purpose.

It's a slightly simplified explanation of our physiology but it drives home a really important point that I want to share with you, as it really ties in with your health and wellbeing.

Here's what Dan says about the three brains:

The "Reptile" brain is simply designed to keep us alive: it sees the world as a dangerous place and is mainly driven by survival instincts and a good amount of stress.

The "Monkey" brain is the more functional part of the brain: it sees the world as a set of challenges to play with while you ride the emotional highs and lows they make you feel.

The "Empire Builder" brain has you see the world as a deeply connected place that you can transform in a meaningful way.

He then proceeds to warn us: "Don't let the reptile run your life". I will add to that by saying: Don't let the reptile run your eating.

Many very brilliant business owners we meet and work with have done such incredible self-development work; they know how to use the more evolved part of their brain, the Empire Builder brain, when it comes to their work. When it comes to food however, they still eat like a reptile. I can assure you that for as long as you "feed your reptile", you will struggle with food.

The reptile fears scarcity above all else. The reptile doesn't think about the big picture. The reptile doesn't think logically or strategically: it simply seeks out what's good for immediate survival and what takes the least amount of energy to obtain.

These are some of the eating habits and patterns that the reptile displays:

- It panics as soon as hunger sets in, fearing that it may lead to starvation.
- It eats whatever is in sight without any plans or strategic thinking.
- It chooses the foods that give the most amount of pleasure with the least amount of effort (highly processed, high in fats and refined sugars, fast food, takeaways.)
- It doesn't stop eating when it's full: since he fears scarcity above all else, it wants to pack in as much as possible now because there may not be enough going around later, so it tends to only stop once all the food is gone.
- It eats fast. Like super fast. It fears that something may come along to steal its food so it packs it in at the speed of light to prevent that from happening.

The reptile doesn't care about your greater goals and aspirations, it only cares about surviving another day. The reptile can't handle plans, strategy, forward thinking: it doesn't care about the big picture. It doesn't care whether you will die prematurely if you continue eating this way, simply because it can't think that far ahead. The reptile still thinks we're living in the wild and in the wild some of these traits were absolutely necessary for our survival: there's no supermarkets in the wild, or fridge/freezers. There's no restaurants, takeaways, not even kitchens.

You don't live in the wild any longer so you must stop eating as if you did. For as long as you let the reptile run your eating, you will NEVER be able to achieve your greatest level of health, fitness and wellbeing.

The monkey brain likes a good old routine. It's purely functional and doesn't like to rock the boat. It just goes for what it knows without questioning it and likes activities that stimulate peak emotions: like feeling too full, getting drunk, the coffee high, the sugar rush.

Here are some eating patterns that the monkey displays:

- It eats what it always has eaten even though it may not be good for it. It doesn't like change. It doesn't like anyone to question its eating routine ("this is what I've always eaten" "this is what we eat in my family" "this is what we eat where I'm from", it claims with conviction.)

- It eats only what is accepted as the norm. It likes to fit in. It eats what its friends eat because if they eat it, it must be good.

- It grazes mindlessly and uses food to entertain itself when bored or in need of a distraction. It loves finger food and to sit in front of the TV going through entire bowls of popcorns, packets of crisps, packs of trail mix. This is just because it likes how the food feels in its mouth and the sensations it's getting from it.

- It cleans its plate and often even other people's plates, not because it's starving but simply because the food is there and therefore should be eaten. It may use the old excuse of "I don't like to waste food" to justify such behavior.

- It is kind of addicted to certain foods, even though it won't call it an addiction, it will call it a "routine" or "habit". "that's just what works for me", it says, even though it may blatantly NOT be working for it at all.

- It spends the day looking forward to consuming the foods it is addicted to: "can't wait to get home to eat that cake, drink that wine, polish that cheese off."

- It uses food or drinks as rewards: "I've worked so hard today: I deserve this bottle of wine and cheese on crackers."

It is possible to generally eat "like a monkey" without causing any major damage. If you have a healthy routine, your monkey will have you stick with it without questioning it, which can actually serve you well. If you however realize that the way you're currently eating doesn't serve your greatest goals and aspirations, the monkey won't be able to help you change that and may actually get in the way because it doesn't like change or disruption AT ALL. For as long as you only feed your Monkey, you're at risk of stagnating and not making progress.

Anyone who wants to transform their health and wellbeing and profoundly improve their eating habits is gonna need to tap into the Empire Builder brain. The Empire Builder only ever has the big picture in mind. It is logical, reasonable and thinks "big". It is wise. Very wise. It doesn't worry about surviving another day because it is too busy thinking about how to change the world. It loves life and all living beings in this world. Its favorite emotional states are the high frequency ones like empathy, gratitude, universal love, joy, compassion.

Here are some eating patterns the Empire Builder displays:

- Forgets to eat lunch and doesn't panic: it simply realizes that it was so present with whatever it was doing, that it didn't want to break the flow by going on lunch break.

- It NEVER eats when he's not hungry. I mean, why would you? It makes no sense to it.

- It NEVER thinks about food unless it is hungry. It has better stuff on its mind (i.e.: changing the world.)

- It doesn't live to eat, mainly eats to live. Mostly sees food as fuel rather than rewards, escape etc.

- It generally doesn't eat food it doesn't like unless there's truly no other option at all. if possible, It would rather wait until it can get something that works for it.

- It doesn't eat food that doesn't make it feel good: the point of eating when hungry is to feel better afterwards, not worse.

- It doesn't eat food that "saps" its energy and makes it feel heavy and drained: again, energy efficiency is its upmost priority.

- It doesn't eat food that takes a very long time to digest and process because it needs that energy for other vital tasks (did I mention, it wants to change the world?)

- It doesn't eat food that it knows doesn't serve its greater goals and aspirations. It is not even tempted by it because the big picture is more important to it than a momentary pleasure.

The Empire builder wants to feel vibrant, light, vital and full of energy so that It can easily tap into the emotional states that it loves the most. It prefers foods that give him high quality, slow-release energy. It doesn't like the high and lows of food addictions and cravings because they pull energy away from the important stuff. It doesn't like to feel too full. It doesn't panic about food. It doesn't crave food: it craves empathy, joy, universal love and compassion.

The most effective eating routine is one that has the greater purpose of the Empire Builder in mind but at the same time doesn't allow the reptile to kick in. It then leverages on the Monkey's love for repeatable tasks to maintain it.

11 tips to eat like an Empire Builder:

1. Avoid skipping meals when hungry: although the Empire Builder doesn't have a problem with this, you may put yourself at risk of a "reptile attack", where you feel so hungry you end up eating anything in sight.

2. Take regular breaks throughout your meals to put the utensils down and become present with the act of eating. Really taste the food. Learn to notice how it feels in your body and how it makes you feel right after. Slow down. There's no rush. Nobody is gonna steal your food from you.

3. Carry healthy snacks with you at all time. Even just an apple, small pack of nuts or cereal bar. This will keep the reptile at bay as you'll feel like you have back up; it will also prevent you from snacking on junk or eating a meal you know doesn't work for you because "you have no choice."

4. If you get to the point where you are very hungry and the reptile has kicked in, it will want you to choose the biggest and most calorie dense food option it can get its hands on. To avoid eating too much of something that will drain you afterwards, build a habit of having a fruit or vegetable starter before you move onto the main course (like an apple and carrot salad with no dressing). Also remind yourself regularly that you are NEVER at risk of dying from starvation. You can start smaller and choose to have more afterwards if you are still really hungry.

5. Drink plenty of water throughout the day and in particular first thing in the morning: thirst can be misdiagnosed as hunger. The Monkey loves it when you make this mistakes because eating is one of its favorite hobbies. Drink a large glass of water before each meal so that you can take care of your thirst before you take care of your hunger.

6. When eating finger foods (popcorns, trailmix, nuts, seeds, olives, pretzels) always go for single portion sizes rather than eating from a large bag: it's so easy for the Monkey to take over and have you eat a whole 500gram pack of almonds when really, all you needed to tie you over was a small handful.

7. As much as possible, avoid foods that over stimulate your dopamine centers and cause massive sugar-highs which will therefore lead to massive crashes: the monkey loves to ride that roller coaster endlessly.

8. Avoid eating when distracted. Build a routine of taking a meal break to focus fully on your eating and nothing else (no TV, computer, phone, work, arguments). This will allow you to stay in touch with the physical sensations, avoid over eating and learn to distinguish which food works best for you and why.

9. Avoid eating when you're not hungry: contrary to popular belief, you will actually be more prone to overeating because, if you weren't hungry to begin with, how are you going to know when you've had enough? Also, the digestive process is the second most energy-expensive processes for the body so eating when not hungry won't give you more energy, it will actually take energy away from you.

10. Plan ahead. Learn to identify the foods that work best for you and that make you feel your best at all times and set yourself up for success by having them handy and readily available to you as much as possible. Doing a one week food log every month or quarter may help with this. Make sure you don't just log all your food but also, most importantly, how the food made you feel afterwards

11. Avoid eating food that you don't need or that doesn't make you feel good, unless you absolutely have no other choice (which is actually way less likely to ever happen than you may think). The fear of "wasting" food may kick in at this point. Remind yourself that eating something that doesn't serve you is the worst form of waste there is because nobody will benefit and only you will suffer: YOU ARE NOT THE BIN!

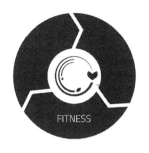

FITNESS

CHAPTER 5

Fitness

Our bodies are designed to move. This is a reality we can't escape: there's no shortcut around this fact, or magic pill that can deliver the same positive effects of regular exercise. Your greatest level of health, fitness and overall life satisfaction will continue to escape you, if you don't make an effort to establish a fitness routine and deeply embed it in your day to day life.

This is because, as previously mentioned, our bodies have evolved through millions of years of living in the wild where regular physical activity was necessary for our survival. Our modern and sedentary lives are therefore not only quite unnatural to our bodies but also very new to us, in the big scheme of things. Our lifestyle is often not conducive to our peak performance.

The benefits of exercise have long since been tried and tested and range from the purely physical (weight loss, improved muscle tone and bone density, decreased risk of chronic disease, improved skin health and lung function), to the emotional and psychological (increased energy levels and relaxation, improved quality of sleep, better moods).

Most busy professionals get to the end of the day feeling too drained and exhausted to work out when sadly, working out would be the very thing that would make them feel more energized and allow them to rest better after a long day at work.

Regular exercise also helps with weight loss in more ways than simply burning more calories: increasing your muscle mass and tone will not only make you look leaner but will also increase your resting metabolic rate, since muscles use more calories than fat. Studies also show that exercise also helps regulate the hormones in charge of appetite and satiety, resulting in less hunger overall.

With all that said, it is important to clarify that regular exercise shouldn't be mistaken for "going to the gym". You can and should make an effort to discover the ways that work best for you and that you actually enjoy. No point trying to commit to running a marathon if you hate running and if it causes more pain (physical or physiological) than pleasure. The only thing to bear in mind, when building a weekly routine, is that it should include all three pillars of wholistic physical fitness (read on for more details) but how you go about this is entirely up to you.

It is also very important to bear in mind that, especially when starting off or getting back into it after a long break, you should be realistic in your expectations of what your body can handle. Slowly, gradually increase the length and intensity of your workouts only once you genuinely feel that you've mastered whatever level you're on.

This will allow you to prevent injuries but most importantly it will make it so that you don't hate the process. Of course it's important to challenge yourself, get out of your comfort zone and test boundaries, however you're WAY more likely to stick long term with something you enjoy and feel that you're actually getting better at. I'll never get tired of reminding our shifters that Success is our greatest motivator: feeling like we're doing good and actually improving will spur us on WAY more than feeling we're failing miserably and struggling every moment along the way.

We tend to have this counterproductive association with exercise whereby if it doesn't hurt, it's not good enough. If it's not "too hard" we won't be getting any results. If it doesn't leave us crawling and shattered, it doesn't count as a decent workout. It's simply not true. The most comprehensive lifestyle population study ever done, called the Blue Zone study, shows that the fittest people on heart all have many healthy lifestyle factors in common such as regular exercise; however none of those people actually go to the gym!

Their usual forms of regular exercise range from gardening, to walking/hiking etc. No HIIT training, Cross-fit or Power Yoga in sight.

Don't get me wrong, I have nothing against the gym or any of the modern forms of exercise and practice some of them regularly myself; the point I want to convey is that there is no one-size-fit-all approach and very often, less is more. Consistency is more important than intensity so finding something that you love and can stick to in the long run will ALWAYS beat killing yourself the odd time here or there, and then taking days to recover and build up the courage to go back at it.

So keep it real, keep it enjoyable, keep it consistent and last but not least, keep is balanced by integrating all three main pillars of wholistic fitness: Cardio, Flexibility and Strength.

Cardio

Cardiovascular fitness is fundamental to good health. You can be as strong as an Ox but if you can't run for the bus or climb a flight of stairs without feeling like your heart may explode in your chest, you will not feel like your best self because you won't be your best self.

Imaging living in the wild again, where our bodies are truly meant to live and designed to survive: every single activity out there would require a great deal of cardiovascular fitness. From hunting and gathering food, to fetching water, to escaping predators by literally running for your life: all these activities require (and therefore encourage) great functioning of the heart, arteries, veins and lungs.

Our bodies are designed to move. It is in our DNA. We are designed to live active lifestyles and have done so for WAY longer than we've been living the sedentary lives of the modern age. Cardiovascular activity is not optional. It is a fundamental part of a wholistic and healthy routine that should not be skipped.

Some of the most obvious benefits of Cardio activities are:

- strengthening the heart (which is not only an organ but also a muscle)
- improving blood circulation and therefore lowering blood pressure
- improving lung capacity, therefore reducing asthma symptoms
- regulating weight and aiding weight loss where needed

However there are tons more benefits that are less commonly known, such as:

- improving the quality of your sleep (by helping regulate hormone levels)
- strengthening your immune system (by increasing anti-bodies in the blood)
- improving brain power (by reducing loss of tissue generally caused by aging)
- boosting your mood (by regulating hormones)
- decreasing the risk of falls (by improving balance and agility)

Again I feel compelled to specify that it doesn't mean you must be able to run marathons or have to hit the treadmill every single day. Running is not the only way to practice cardio and could, in many instances, be the least advisable.

One very common mistake we see happen time and again is individuals who have never exercised or haven't done so in a long time who, out of the blue (usually on January 2nd or 3rd), decide to put on their trainers and head out for a life changing 10 mile run because they need to "do some cardio".

Not only do they generally tend to have an horrendous time, for obvious reasons, but also many of them end up incurring injuries that quickly dampen this flicker of good will, giving them the perfect excuse to give up before they could experience any long term benefits.

Cardio is great. Running may or may not be. If you want to start building a cardio routine or get back on it after a long break, you HAVE to start very small and gentle. Even smaller and gentler than you would think.

Here's a list of more gentle activities that can help you get started gradually and mindfully:

1. **Brisk walking:** pick up a pace that's faster than a casual stroll but that you can sustain for a good 5-10 consecutive minutes. Then slow down for a few minutes, and pick it up again. Just 15 minutes of this a day, 3-5 times a week would be a good place to start from, for someone who's brand new to any cardio activity. You can then progressively extend the length of the brisk walking and decrease the amount of rest time to shift up a gear, whenever you feel you're ready for it.

2. **Swimming:** possibly one of the best forms of cardio as the water massively reduces the impact on joints and ligaments. Swimming is so effective because it's very therapeutic for the body and the mind. When you swim, you're generally completely switched off from distractions such as technology and any other stimuli from the environment. This will allow you to work the body whilst resting the mind through only concentrating it on the task at hand (for the most part).

3. **Cycling:** slightly less impact than running, this can be a great option if one is really careful about safety, especially when cycling on the streets amongst cars. Many people choose it as a mean of transport too, which means that you save time, money and workout out whilst getting places: it doesn't get more efficient than that!

4. **Playing sports (soccer, football, tennis etc.):** this is often underestimated in these days as we've lost touch with the idea of "having fun" as a mean of working out. We also tend to put too much pressure on ourselves and easily get caught up in the "performance" aspect rather than the fun aspect. Especially those of us who have past experiences in professional or semi-professional sports. The point is not to win. The point is to MOVE. That's all that truly matters.

5. **Yoga:** tends to be considered purely a stretching activity but many yoga practices are actually also incredibly good for cardio. From Bikram to Power, Vinyasa, Ashtanga and many more, there's so much on offer these days and most of them will actually prove to be fantastic cardio sessions without carrying the risks and heavy impact of other disciplines such as running, cycling or playing sport. Not to mention the added benefit of a practice that incentives mindfulness by encouraging mind-body connection. Yoga can truly be the ultimate game-changer.

6. **Cleaning or gardening:** anything that moves your body, elevates your heart rate and shortens your breath for a considerable amount of time counts as a cardio activity. And I truly mean anything!

7. **Dancing:** This is one of my favorite "unusual" cardio options and one that has often saved the day on occasions when I did NOT feel like working out AT ALL. Yes, it happens to all of us. Including the professionals. It will never stop happening. The way I counteract those moments is to put on my favorite fast song and dance to my heart's content until the end. I often have told myself

that I would only dance to one song and ended up doing a full workout afterwards as dancing gave me the kick and stimuli I needed to get going; just think of it this way. It can be hard to push a huge ball into motion but once it gets going, it will be even harder to stop ;)

8. **Climbing stairs:** one thing anyone can do right away to get more active is to climb stairs at any given opportunity throughout the day. Remember that the small stuff, done daily, adds up to bring new results so NEVER underestimate small new actions but also, don't get impatient when expecting the results. Instead learn to embrace and enjoy the act itself and have fun with it, just like kids do when they climb.

The essence I'd love to leave you with is that there is no such thing as the perfect cardio activity. In fact, the perfect one is the one you actually enjoy most and are most likely to stick with regularly (at least 3 times a week) and for the long run (at least 100 years!). Whatever that is: start now, have fun and never give up!

Flexibility

Being flexible is grossly undervalued, tightness however, especially when chronic, can be quite debilitating and even harmful. My husband runs a very successful therapeutic massage practice and most ailments he treats are back, neck and shoulder pain due to chronic tension and tightness.

Our sedentary lives are unnatural for our bodies and the daily use (or even abuse, quite often) of technology cause us to maintain unhealthy postures for very long periods of time.

We spend too much time sitting down when our bodies are not even designed to sit on chairs at all, rather we're meant to be sitting on the floor; this leads to chronic tightness of the hips, hamstrings and lower back.

We're also constantly hunching forward, looking at phone screens, computers or even driving: we never bend backwards to counteract this constant forward bending and this leads to constant strain on our neck and shoulders.

And even those of us who are active often underestimate the importance of stretching and therapeutic practices such as restorative (AKA Yin) yoga, Body Wheel Therapy®, Therapeutic massage, Chiro-practice, Stretching, Foam Rolling.

One can easily get hooked on high intensity practices such as Hot yoga, HIIT, CrossFit, running and before you know it, we skip the stretching before and after or neglect a slower pace class because we're constantly chasing the "adrenaline high".

Doing too much of one thing, even a small thing or a good thing, can be detrimental if we don't balance it out; we constantly have to emphasize this with our clients who are generally high achievers and find it hard to slow down their tempo.

There's also a gross and diffused misconception that therapeutic practices are only for injury recovery or for those who lack mobility or stamina. Many of us wait to get an injury before finally giving the body some time to recover when in fact, embedding therapeutic practices and stretches in your weekly routine is exactly what you need to do to prevent the injury altogether.

Let me reinforce once more how important it is to view your wellbeing from a wholistic perspective: so long as you focus all your time, energy and effort on one thing only, your greatest level of health, fitness and mind-body confidence will forever escape you. You can be the strongest man on earth but if you can't scratch your back, you will still not be your most functional self. Much the same, you can be the fastest man on heart, but if your hamstrings are so tight that they constantly pull on your hips and lower back, you'll still be living your (fast) life in pain.

Most people complain to us that they just "don't have the time" to stretch after a workout or go to yoga: I routinely remind them that I don't have the power to add hours to their day (that would surely be quite a popular gift), I do however have the ability of helping them allocate their time more effectively so that whatever time they spend exercising in a week is well balanced to maximize results whilst also preventing injuries and set-backs.

Other benefits of stretching practices are:

- Increased circulation: it improves blood flow to the most remote parts of the body therefore improving the supply of nutrients to muscles and joints. This prevents pain from injury. Some of the tightest joints in the body (hips, knees, ankles) are tight due to lack of blood flow.

- Reduced risk of injury due to tight muscles and ligaments.

- Improved ROM (range of motion), which also leads to less injury and makes you less prone to accidental falling.

- Decreased stress: one of the main side effects of stress on the body is that the tension will cause you to involuntarily contract you muscles. This leads to chronic physical tension and maybe even pain which will in turn lead to more stress. Perfect example of a catch 22. In order to release stress, you could start from the mind by performing breathing or meditation exercises which will allow you to "loosen" the mental tension and will in turn facilitate relaxation in the body. You could just as well start from the body and if fact, if you're not at all used to mindfulness practices, this may be easier and therefore more effective. By perfuming activities that relax the body and allow you to "loosen up" the physical tension, you will find yourself more able to release the mental tension and stress.

- Prevents Headaches and Migraines: anyone that suffers from these regularly knows all too well how debilitating they can be. Some professionals spend days or even weeks recovering from them and live in constant fear of when the next one may show up. Yet, when probed about their wellness routines, they often tells us they simply don't have the time to take better care of themselves. Most headaches and migraines can easily and effectively be prevented by not allowing the tension to build up over time. Stretching practices can be SO beneficial in this instances as, like mentioned before, they often work on a mind-body level.

- Increased strength, endurance and overall athletic performance: Yes, that's right, you will get stronger if you stretch regularly than if you don't. Lengthening you muscles catalyzes faster growth by stimulating them to build denser and stronger fibers.

Remember that, like with everything else, less is more so adjust your weekly routine to introduce some therapeutic practices regularly: even just 3-5 minutes of Body Wheel Therapy ® a day will add up at the end of the week. In general, anything you can realistically stick with for at least 3-5 days is precisely where you should start, as small as it may be. You can even start by just practicing what we call a "micro routine" every day, at least once during or after your workday. Trust me when I say, you will notice incredible results after a few months of regular practice.

To find our more about the Body Wheel Therapy® and it's huge benefits, simply visit **https://www.wholeshiftwellness .com/body-wheel-therapy/**

Strength

For a very long time in my life I held the misconception that I didn't need to be strong in order to be healthy. When I discovered yoga in my late twenties, I really felt like I'd finally found the thing that worked best for me. Yoga allowed me to work my body and my mind at the same time: it transformed my body in ways that I could have never imagined. It transformed my approach to life as a whole, in greater ways than I could have hoped for.

For many years from then, I genuinely believed that I didn't need anything more than yoga in order to be healthy and happy. I've now grown to believe that, as much as many yoga practices are truly some of the most wholistic forms of exercise out there, a lot has to be said for complementing them with other activities that build your strength in other ways.

Meeting my husband was pivotal to this shift in mindset: he's not only an incredible yoga practitioner (and silver medalist at the USA yoga asana championships), but also a passionate fan of weight training and former semi-professional body builder. He is a true embodiment and proof that we don't have to choose between being strong and flexible and actually, our greatest level of health, fitness and wellbeing is acquired once we learn to develop ALL three pillars of physical fitness simultaneously. This inevitably has to include some weight training.

The same disclaimer applies here as it does to the cardio section: weight training does NOT have to involve going to the gym. I haven't been to the gym in many years and only ever go when I'm on holiday. Any other time of the year, I practice quick and effective routines in the comfort of my home and only need two small sets of dumbbells and four small sets of ankle weights.

There are several different school of thought when it comes to weight training, especially for women: some advocate limiting the weights used in order to avoid "bulking up" whilst others believe that a great shape can be achieved by ladies through lifting heavy weights since our muscles can only ever naturally grow so much anyway.

I'm not a huge advocate of either and actually believe that much of it comes to personal preference: lifting heavy weights definitely requires going to the gym, unless one can afford building an in-home gym. This means that those who are not fans of the gym environment as a whole are going to forever be put off from doing it. Other people love the gym and the look that heavy weight lifting allows them to acquire, therefore they would never feel completely fulfilled by light-weight, in-home routines. In essence, you've got to find what works for you and go for it.

There are a number of benefits that come from lifting weights: such benefits are very hard, if not impossible to get from only practicing callisthenic routines.

Here are some of them:

- **Increase in muscle mass:** as the body ages, it has a tendency to lose muscle mass (a process known as sarcopenia). Lifting weights helps prevent this.
- **Body fat Loss:** More muscle mass also means a more toned look and an increase in your metabolic rate which will in turn reduce your fat storages by increasing your energy requirements even when at rest.

- **Improved balance:** An increase in muscle mass is also related to better balance and less risk of falls since larger and denser muscles are more stable.

- **Improved daily functioning:** Larger muscle mass will also help you perform ALL daily activities more efficiently and effectively, especially those that require coordination.

- **Better posture:** Stronger muscles will certainly improve your posture and stance. This is obviously great for preventing chronic tightness and pain and I just can't stress enough the importance of not settling for a life riddled with pain.

- **Increase in bone strength:** lifting weights will allow you to increase your bone density, which is particularly relevant to women who are more likely to experience a loss in bone density (also known as osteoporosis) as they age. Stronger bones are less likely to break so this will lead to a decreased risk of fractures.

- **There is also another more subtle but very powerful side effect that comes from developing your strength:** it is one that has less to do with your body and more to you with your Mind-body, as we call it. I experienced it firsthand myself when I finally got inspired by my husband and started working out with weights for the first time in my life. What I realized is that by getting stronger I was not only improving my posture but also, more importantly, my stance and with that came an incredible and unexpected boost in overall Mind-body confidence. Take a minute to think about and analyze the stance of the most confident people you know in life. Chances are, you'll find they all have one thing in common: great posture combined with a powerful stance. They're not hunching forward, hiding themselves from the world, instead they stand tall, proud and powerful. They exude strength and let me tell you, it is very hard to exude strength when you're not feeling strong in your body.

Working out at the gym tests your comfort zone and puts you firmly in touch with your body's full power and potential and there's a lot of mental power that comes from that. It's like driving a very powerful car that you know can go very fast. Or a 4x4 you know can handle any terrain. You'll get on the road with an extra spring in your step, confident that you'll be strong enough to face anything that life will throw at you throughout the day. For sure physical strength is not the only or most important kind of strength one should develop but it sure does matter and should not be neglected.

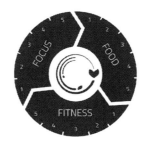

CHAPTER 6

5Ms To Success

Exercise:

List three to five qualities that you believe allow people to stick to their wellness routines, reach their goals and maintain them in the long run:

1. _____

2. _____

3. _____

4. _____

5. _____

Our work transforming the health and wellbeing of over 500 leaders across 5 countries has allowed us to gain a wealth of experience. We've learnt a lot not only from our own individual wellness journeys but also from being exposed to the unique challenges and breakthroughs our shifters experienced on the road to their most fit, healthy and confident selves.

As a result of this experience, we are able to clearly identify the most common mistakes busy professionals encounter time and time again when making such shifts. These mistakes transcend geography, since we've seen them happen across 5 countries. They also transcend gender, ethnicity, profession and even age, to some extent. We see them happen all the time and have noticed how massively they can impact the success rate and achievements of even the most determined individuals out there.

Our unique 5 steps methodology was developed as a direct result of these findings: we saw how much quicker our shifters were able to achieve not just changes, but actual profound transformations once we worked with them to avoid these very common yet stubborn hurdles and roadblocks.

It was as if they'd been driving with the handbrake on the entire time and all of a sudden, once they released the break, they were able to reach full speed, fulfill their greatest potential (greater than they could even imagine) and get to a destination that was even further than what they set out to accomplish.

It took us over 20+ years to acquire all the knowledge and experience we've now distilled in our methodology: wouldn't you like to cut through the chase and get to the point in a friction of the time?

Many people take years and years trying to figure out the journey on their own, jumping from short cut to short cut, from fad to trend, hoping that this would finally be the miracle pill (or diet, or machine) that will deliver the results they're so desperate to achieve: once they make up their mind that it's time to go after their goals, they simply can't wait to get there and fall prey to all the short term fixes that are out there these days.

I would be lying to you if I told you that I never made that mistake myself: I've tried every single "diet" and regimen under sun to no avail. In fact, every attempt to go about it the "fast" way, would end up setting me back months if not years. I even had to go through a long break in my life where I completely stopped any attempt to lose weight and get healthier just to give my mind and body a break from the endless rollercoaster of diet on/diet off. I was lucky enough to have the clear realization one day that my choices were just making matters worse.

Every time I decided that "this is the year I'm gonna get the body of my dreams", the inevitable would ensue: I would set up the most extreme regimen, look for the latest fad diet, sign up to some intense class and commit to a life that had absolutely not even a shred of fun in it because surely, you can't have fun AND be fit and healthy, right? Not if you want to get there fast!

Inevitably (and quite predictably), such plans never lasted. Sure, I had "good spells" when I was able to stick with it for months, at times even years, but sooner or later, something small would happen that would throw me off course and before I knew it, I would be ALL into self-sabotaging mode: eating all the things I'd felt so deprived of for so many days or even months, lazing around, going out for endless drinks with the friends I had neglected the entire time I was trying to "be good". Some would call it "having fun".

The fundamental problem was that I thought of wellness as something you have to endure: something generally unpleasant that you must stick to with sheer willpower. I had no idea how to live a life you love AND be in the best shape of my life. Our shifters generally come to us with the same belief system. If only I had a penny for every time someone told me that they "lack will-power" and that's why they're unfit and unhealthy!

In fact, I wouldn't be surprised if you listed will power as one of the traits that allow people to stick to their goals. Let me tell you, I use close to NO willpower now and I'm by and far in the best shape of my life. The years when I was relying on willpower to get me to my goals, were the years I was struggling most.

Think of willpower as a muscle: if you keep using it and using it and using it, it will sooner or later give up on you. Those who succeed only use willpower in case of emergency. What you need to succeed is a strategy, a proven methodology that will set you up for success as much and as often as possible, so that you don't have to rely on willpower the whole time.

You also need to accept and appreciate that the journey of trans-formation is likely to take longer than you'd like. Maybe even three times longer. However I can guarantee you that It will be a MUCH faster journey than wasting 20 years on fads, diets and magic pills than don't work.

Temporary change will NEVER facilitate profound transforma-tion: lifestyle change will. Lifestyle change takes time but more importantly it takes strategy. You can't simply change what you do: you have to transform who you are at the root level so that you get to the point whereby your new healthier habits are not simply something you're doing for a while to get where you want to be; they are actually an extension of who you are.

Here are the 5 essential steps we know will take you there for good.

Move Gradually

Every single professional we work with underestimates the power of compound interests when it comes to health and wellbeing. They're so constantly brainwashed with the latest marketing ploy around some short term fix that they find it very hard to accept this truly is the journey of a lifetime.

We've seen professionals struggle for decades to get a handle over their fitness (physical and mental) and nutrition. Yet when we encourage them to think of changing their habits over a period of at least 6 months to a year, they all get a bit unsettled and wonder why it would "take so long".

I may have said this before but stop and think for a moment at all the time you've wasted on short term fixes and diets that didn't work or only worked temporarily. Chances are, it will amount to months if not years. The journey to your most fit, healthy and confident self is not a journey of quick change: it is a journey of profound transformation from the inside out. What is the difference between change and transformation, you may ask? Change can happen very quickly but is also easily reversible. Transformation on the other hand may take longer but once you have it, it's yours for the rest of your life. A butterfly could never, ever go back to being a caterpillar.

You've got to Move Gradually along the way in order to give enough time to each new habit to sink into your consciousness and become second nature, much like brushing your teeth or taking a shower. Only once a habit is truly embedded into your daily or weekly routine, should you then work to establish another, or work to take the existing habit to a new level. It's like building a new house from the ground up: each new brick lays perfectly on top of the previous one and so on but if you layer the bricks too quickly without giving time for the cement and glue between them to dry, sooner or later the whole structure will crumble down, no matter how high you managed to get it.

I invite you to resist the temptation to rush through the process: rushing is a sign that you're not truly embracing it, instead you're merely enduring it in the hope that it will get you to your goals. It may also be a sign that your plan is not working for you and needs tweaking. The problem with enduring is that it's generally not enjoyable or sustainable. The moment you get yourself in "endurance" mode, you're out of the present moment and only focused on the goal you're trying to achieve. However, please think: are you going to maintain a goal if you hated the journey that got you there? Aren't you more likely to maintain a goal if you actually enjoyed the process of achieving it, for the most part?

Don't get me wrong, using your goals as motivation is a fundamental part of the journey but only if done in a smart way. Let me give you an example: you can use your goal to motivate you in doing a workout that you don't initially feel like doing; you know all too well that you simply need that initial push and once you get going, you will actually enjoy the process and will be glad to have done it. This only works however if your workout is carefully tailored to your level so that it pushes you but not is such way that actually feels unbearable and uncomfortable or even painful for the duration. If it does, you'll resist it no matter how great your goal is and how much you want it.

Pushing yourself out of your comfort zone is necessary but can be counterproductive if you don't do it in a smart way. Moving gradually ensures that you're not setting the bar so high that you either always feel like you're never going to achieve it or it feels too painful to get it done each time.

Take your time. Pace yourself. What's a year or even two or three in the big scheme of your life as a whole? Only the habits you stick to in the long run will bring forth the profound transformation you're after. Sure, you can have minor "rev the engine" moments when you take things to the next level but you've got to be smart in giving yourself time to digest each phase before you move to the next. Let that glue dry out fully before you stack new bricks on top of the old. Do whatever you need to do to enjoy the process as much as possible. Resist the temptation to rush.

Every time you get eager and look for a short term fix, you're likely to burn yourself out and end up giving up, and every time you give up, you lose momentum and end up making it so much harder for yourself to get going again. Remember that nobody likes to fail. Success is your greatest motivation. You will leverage on your successes WAY more than your failures so the more you can set yourself up for success, the more likely you are to get to your destination. Slow and steady truly wins this race.

Move Gradually and I assure you that you'll get there much faster than you can even imagine: you may even get to the point that you'll be so present and absorbed in the daily routines you actually enjoy, that you'll stop paying so much attention to the end goal and that's precisely when it'll appear before your eyes and surprise you beyond your expectations.

Life only happens in the present moment. Use your goals in a smart way: stop living for the future of your dreams and start creating the present of your dreams. That's when you'll unlock WAY greater joy than you ever thought possible.

Motivate Yourself

We tend to underestimate the importance of constantly reminding ourselves of your deepest motivations and highest goals, especially when it comes to our health and wellbeing. We think we know them and completely take for granted the process of delving deep into them to unpack them and bring them to light. Motivation is less of a gift and more of a trained skill.

We're all motivated on January 3rd, when we're benefiting from the momentum of the New Year and the holiday indulgences that weigh heavy on us (pun intended), but why do many lose that motivation only a few weeks, or even days into it? Because we fail to unpack that motivation in its deepest layers and then reinforce it regularly. Daily even.

The main difference between individuals who don't give up on their dreams, and those who do, is often their level of motivation. The great news is that you can practice motivation and get progressively better at it until you'll get to a point where nothing will take you off your chosen path This is a small yet powerful distinction that will make a HUGE difference in all areas of your life.

We've all had motivating experiences in our lives: we've all watched a movie that has inspired us or read a book that has given us some awesome juice, met a person that has lifted our spirits or watched a video that has inspired us to transform our lives. These instances are very important to spark profound transformation, however they're not sufficient to keep you charged for the whole journey. You must always leverage on an injection of motivation by creating a long term plan of action around it.

There's nothing wrong with using the momentum of the New Year resolutions to set some new goals and routines, however it is important to remember that the New Year fever only lasts a few days, whereas profound transformation takes months if not years to achieve.

Imagine your greatest level of health, fitness and wellbeing as a tree: that gush of motivation you get at the beginning of a new year is simply pushing the seed of your beautiful tree into the ground but not that deep into the ground; just a few inches down, which actually is enough for the seed to sprout. In order for that little first plant to grow into the beautiful tree that represent your greatest self, it must develop very strong and deep roots. The deeper the roots, the more able it will be to withstand the elements which inevitably, sooner or later, will shake it about and risk un-rooting it.

At the beginning, when the seedling is only a little plant and doesn't yet have strong roots, it needs A LOT of protection from the elements. Having a routine that constantly reinforces your motivation is one of the strongest protections against the elements such as parties, unsupportive friends and family, trips and any unforeseen circumstances that are bound to show up.

You simply cannot motivate yourself enough, especially at the beginning of the journey to your most fit, healthy and confident self: that's why those who choose to outsource their accountability and work with a trainer or coach are more likely to succeed. By paying someone to constantly reinforce your motivation, you will be WAY less likely to run out of it. Not to mention, you'll have the extra and very powerful motivation of not wanting to waste the money you've invested on it.

In the first few months or even years, your motivation routine has to be your number one priority: it needs to be consistent and repetitive. You've got to delve deep into your goals and become present with the pros and cons that come with them. You've got to remind yourself of these pros and cons every single day. I repeat: EVERY.SINGLE.DAY. The moment you get relaxed or bored of this repetition and start taking it for granted, you will be at risk of a storm uprooting your little plant and trust me when I say: there will be plenty of storms coming your way. That's how life is.

I've been doing this kind of work for over a decade now and even I have a solid motivating routine that keeps me in touch with my ever growing and expanding goals. There will never come a time when you no longer need a motivating routine. Never. But there will come a time when your routine is so embedded in you that it won't feel like a burden or a task you tick off. It will be almost second nature and it won't take as long as it did when you first started. You may however need to regularly upgrade it to match your level of growth and development.

Here are some useful tips to create an effective motivation strategy and routine that will work:

1. **Use pen on paper:** write down your goals on a journal. The act of writing down has very powerful effects on the brain that you simply don't get from only thinking about things in your head or even talking about them with someone. Put pen to paper before you do anything else.

2. **Dig deep:** don't just identify your goals, dig deep into why they matter to you (see the 5 Whys exercise earlier in the book) and how your life will look like in 3-5-10 years if you achieve them versus what it would look like

if you don't. Remember, the deeper your roots, the stronger your tree, so the deeper you dig into your subconscious mind and discover what pleasures and fears really move you, the stronger you'll be.

3. **Read them daily:** you've got to have your goals up somewhere where you can see them every, single, day. Ideally more than one place. It's true that you'll eventually get used to seeing them and feel like you're noticing them less but your subconscious mind will still pick them up every time you just glance at them. You can even set them as reminders on your phone every day/week.

4. **Share them:** not only with the people you love and care about but also with anyone who you spend a lot of time with regularly. The only side note for this is to choose wisely who you share them with (more on this later on) so start with the most supportive of your family, friends and colleague and enroll them into keeping you accountable if/when needed. Human beings are not naturally self-motivated: we need people outside of ourselves to keep us going. This is basic human nature and nothing to be ashamed of so create a support system as that'll make ALL the difference in the long haul.

5. **Review and update:** remember that as you progress, you will grow and expand so something that motivates you right now may not work later on. Your goals are not set in stone, they're fluid sign posts and should work for you before you work for them. Set a reminder to review them at least every 6 months and see what may need upgrading.

Manage Your Thoughts

Another thing we often forget we're in control of is our thoughts. By this I don't necessarily mean that you can control every single thought that comes up in your mind, that's impossible. However you can certainly control which thoughts you give time and attention to, and whether or how you react to your thoughts.

Most of our clients tell us how they struggle to handle those moments when they just "can't be bothered to exercise" or "can't resist the temptation to eat a whole cake or drink a whole bottle of wine".

Most people believe that those of us who generally stick to our healthy habits never have those moments of temptation or lack of motivation. I still have days when I don't feel like working out. Every week in fact. For sure, they don't happen as often as they did when I first embarked on the journey of self-improvement but they still happen.

Here's the thing, the more practiced you become at implementing your wellness routine, the more it will become second nature and you'll actually enjoy doing it more than not doing it, but this takes quite a bit of practice and, especially at the beginning, you'll have plenty of moments when it won't feel like much fun at all.

That's when the practice of managing your thoughts will come in handy.

What do I mean by managing your thoughts, you may wonder? Here's the thing: every time you skip a workout you had planned or eat and drink something you know is not conducive to your goals, there's a little voice in your head that makes up a reason or excuse as to why that's a better idea than sticking to your habits. Have you ever paid attention to what this little voice tells you? Many people don't pay attention to this voice but, even worse, they identify with it and end up doing what it says without question.

Please remember: that voice in your head is not you. That's your self-sabotaging voice: it gets in your way time and time again, and the more you listen to it and do as it says, the more you strengthen its hold on you. Giving into your self-sabotaging thoughts is a habit as much as NOT giving into them is: whichever habit you practice the most will simply become the most prominent habit AND it is never too late to learn a new habit.

The first most important thing you can do to start loosening the grip of your self-sabotaging thoughts is to identify them. Like I said, we often don't even recognize them so paying attention is of fundamental importance. Take at least a week if not a month to notice every single time you break your commitment to yourself: what did the voice say in that instance? What did it have you believe to make you do what it said rather than what you had set out to do?

Did it tell you that "just one cookie won't hurt. After all, you've been so good this past week. You deserve to treat yourself!"?

It may have then proceeded to tell you "you've ruined it all by eating that cookie! You're such a failure! You weren't even hungry! You may as well go all out today and start again tomorrow!!"?

Did it tell you that "You're just too tired to work out today. There's no point exercising as you won't be able to give it your best so it would be a waste of time"?

It may have told you that "You've been so good for a whole month and you can hardly see any difference at all! I know Mark from work said you looked good but he's always nice to everyone so that doesn't count. It's obviously not working so you may as well go to the pub, have some fun and get drunk with the guys. Who cares it's a Wednesday, life is meant to be enjoyed and we should have fun as often as possible. Even on a Wednesday!"

These are just a few of the examples we see come up time and time again: we think we're all so unique and different and in many ways we are but you'll be surprise how similar our self-sabotaging beliefs sound! That's because they are NOT us.

My self-sabotaging thoughts generally show themselves whenever I stay up later than 10pm on a weekday: I've learnt to interpret them as a bed time alert! The moment they show up, I know I'm 30 minutes late for bed. They say things like: "You deserve a late night snack, Eugene is having one so you should have one too and enjoy it together." Or "You took yoga class AND worked out. You can have it. I know you prefer to have treats at the weekend but you can make an exception for once."

They also sometimes like to put me off my daily workout by saying things like "you can't work out right now the way you planned. You're in the middle of something and there's no point stopping now. You can always work out late or do two workouts tomorrow". You get the idea I'm sure.

After you've spent some time identifying the most common ones for you, and have listed them all down with pen to paper on your journal (once again, please don't skip the process of writing them down!), you need to create some answers to dismantle them.

For example, if a common one for you is "One cookie won't kill you! You've been so good, you deserve to treat yourself", your answer may be "one cookie often becomes many cookies as I know how these foods are not meant to be eaten in moderation and trigger certain physiological responses that are SO hard to resist. Anyway, it's not about just one cookie: It's about sticking to my commitments to myself and practicing the habit of not giving into you, nasty self-sabotaging thought! I'll plan to have a cookie when I say, not when YOU say! Now F***k O** and let me get on with my life!" For example.

The more you practice the habit of NOT giving into your self-sabotaging thoughts, the more you will become less susceptive to their non-conducive influence. This is NOT to say that you'll get to a point where you will not experience any self-sabotaging thoughts at all: as previously mentioned, the journey is never-ending as you're always growing, so as you progressively test your boundaries and limitations more and more, new limiting beliefs will sprout up and try to get in your way but every time, you'll know what to do to tackle them.

Make Plans

The next fundamental step to set yourself up for success is to plan as much as possible, as often as possible, so that you're never caught unprepared and forced to stray off your chosen path. I really can't emphasize this enough: planning is fundamental, especially to begin with and the more of it you do, the better off you'll be.

Meal Planning is one way of making plans that support your new habits. One thing I should clarify however, is that you've got to make sure that you tailor the nature and amount of planning to your lifestyle, as not everyone genuinely needs or enjoys to prepare every single meal of the week in one day. I know there's plenty of advocates of meal planning which will have you believe that is indispensable: I see plenty of awesome meal planning pictures on Instagram but as cool as they look, they may not be the answer for you.

Many of our clients have experienced setting up unsustainable expectations when it comes to meal planning which ended up backfiring on them rather than supporting them on their journeys.

If you are the kind of person that likes to shop once a week and cook everything in bulk, it may well be the answer for you, but if the sheer thought of it makes you feel overwhelmed and puts you off, then there's plenty of softer ways you can plan to succeed.

There are plenty of basic yet effective tips when it comes to food that you can easily implement in a gradual and sustainable way to make improvements that will actually make a difference. Here are some of my favorite, when it comes to food:

1. **Always carry healthy snacks in your bag:** never be caught out and about when hungry without a healthy option readily available. That's precisely when you're most likely to make a choice you didn't intend to as your self-sabotaging thoughts love the excuse of "I had no alternative" to justify eating some junky snack. Carry an apple or a snack bar or some trail mix or any other non-perishable items to fall back on if and when needed. This especially applies to long road trips, flights and holidays.

2. **Keep healthy snacks in your car and office drawer:** for the same reason as above. It's always better to have more options than less. The office drawer stack is particularly important to prevent unhealthy eating from vending machines and canteens which are still unfortunately some of the worst places to find healthy food. If your colleagues have a tendency of always having unhealthy snacks around or if there's always some birthday cake floating around the office, make sure you have your own better choice to go for when temptation arises.

3. **Always cook double (or more) the amount of what you actually need:** like I said, meal planning can be overwhelming for most as it looks and can be harder than many feel comfortable with. However, one easy way to warm to the approach and phase it into your life is to always make sure you cook more than needed so that you always have left overs for the day after or to freeze. I never, ever cook just one or two portions of anything. Whenever I cook rice or legumes, I always cook the

entire bag. Same for pasta and pasta sauces or stir fried rice. I even make salad in bulk (4 portions instead of 2): as long as you don't add any dressing, it will keep in the fridge for 2-4 days.

4. **Make the most of online shopping and subscription boxes:** many people make the silly mistake of doing their grocery shopping after work, when they're more likely to be exhausted and starving. There is not a worse combination for buying food: you're so much more likely to buy processed quick meals and unhealthy snacks. We don't really go to the supermarket anymore, other than to pick up the odd thing we need urgently. All our groceries are delivered to our house once a week and we have a subscription of organic fruit and vegetables that automatically gets delivered without me even having to do anything (unless I want to change anything from the list). Make the most of these options so you set yourself up for success. Keep it as simple, easy and automated as you can.

5. **Learn how to eat healthy at a restaurant:** some people have mixed opinions on this. Very often they tell me that they like to feel "spontaneous" and just go with the flow when eating out. I'm a big fan of planned spontaneity. We only generally eat out once a week and that's when I allow myself to choose whatever (vegan) meal I feel like. I know that one weekly indulgent meal won't have a negative impact on me, overall. If you eat out more than once a week however, this approach is likely to fail you. If you want to improve your health and wellbeing, you will have to learn how to eat healthily at a restaurant which is trickier than at home but absolutely possible.

6. **Always stock your pantry and freezer with staples for a quick emergency meal:** you grocery deliveries should always include a selection of staples that allow you to put together a meal even if you don't have anything fresh in the fridge. For instance we always have frozen veggies, microwave rice, cooked beans, pasta sauces, dried pasta and noodles. These simple items will allow you to always be able to put something together in under 30 minutes and never have to go for some fast food or ready-made unhealthy meal (unless you plan to, of course).

7. **Discover your favorite healthy meals deliveries:** Although ready meals are generally not as good as home cooked ones, these days there are so many healthy meal delivery options. Our chosen partners are the guys from Plant Pots Kitchen, who cook their amazing plant based meals with only fresh and organic ingredients and freeze them on the spot so that it's virtually the same as eating your own leftovers. Do a little investigation. Try a few different ones until you discover your favorite and maybe even set up a subscription so that you always have some of them in the freezer as back up.

8. **Make a list of healthy meals you enjoy:** there's nothing wrong than being hungry and not knowing what to make. As I said, when you're hungry you're most likely to eat whatever is easier and quicker so make sure you have a list (again, written is better) of your favorite healthy and easy meals that you can peruse when you're feeling stuck. This can be developed over time and regularly updated with new discoveries. Attach it to the fridge if needed.

9. **Every week for four to six weeks, cook one new dish:** a very common mistake we see busy professionals make

time and again is that of changing their eating habits too quickly too soon and then feeling out of depth and overwhelmed. The best way to eat more healthily is to start leveraging on the meals you already eat and love which are naturally healthy or can simply be made healthier. Then, once a week, you can venture out of your comfort zone and try one new healthy dish to see if it works for you. Not all of them will but in a few months you'll have easily discovered half a dozen that do the trick and you can add to your list of favorites.

10. **Create a food shopping list of staple items and keep it on your phone:** this is needed even you do have grocery deliveries set up. It's good to quickly glance at the list of staples to make sure you're not missing any. It's also good to have it handy in case you do need to make an emergency trip to the supermarket. You don't even have to go down the aisles that sell junk. You have your list, you stick to it. Done deal.

Monitor Your Progress

The last fundamental step in staying motivated along the way is to monitor your progress as often as possible. Daily would be ideal but if not, then at least weekly. I know that very often the first things that comes to mind in relation to monitoring your health and wellness progress is getting on the scale to measure your weight.

Here's the thing, monitoring your weight is only one small way you can get this done and it may not even be the best way. There are so many different factors which can impact your weight such as water retention, bowel movement, increase in muscle mass, hormones (especially for us ladies); I really wouldn't recommend weighing yourself any more than once a week.

Your weight can be a great indicator of progress and I'm not advocating sticking your head in the sand if you are overweight just because it hurts to admit it: weighing yourself obsessively however may actually be counterproductive and may cause you to miss other markers that are showing progress.

It's important to monitor and measure a variety of different things, and even more important to notice every single little improvement and every small thing you get right every single day. I will never get tired of reminding you that success is your greatest motivation, so the more you can fuel yourself with it, the better you will do, continuously and progressively.

Once again, I recommend you log this in a journal: nothing works better than putting pen to paper. Every day, or at least every week, note all the major challenges you've faced, how you've handled them, what you need to do differently next time.

But then also notice all the things you did how you intended, as small as they may be.

Notice every single step you took in the right direction. Every time you were tempted to skip a workout or eat a piece of cake but didn't. Every day you woke up feeling a little more energetic than the day before. Every time you felt a little more confident and empowered than you did months or weeks ago. Every time you tried a new food you wouldn't have tried before or did a 5 minute meditation you wouldn't have done before. You truly can't do this enough, especially to begin with. No win is too small to celebrate. No improvement is too little to be acknowledged.

You have to become your biggest fan and marvel at the amazing capabilities of your Mind-body. We take for granted how amazing our Mind-bodies are, what they're capable of doing each day, how much they're able to transform and improve, how quickly they progress. What if we learned to acknowledge and appreciate the most simple of things like waking up each day, being able to walk and climb stairs, type on a keyboard, sit and stand up? Appreciating the small stuff is not only key to staying motivated along your wellness journey but it is actually key to enjoying life to its fullest extent.

Profound transformation happens one little step at a time: we tend to expect and only celebrate the big wins, but those are not the most important nor are they the most transformational. It often takes hundreds if not thousands of little wins and improvements in order for a big win to even be possible.

Think about little babies when they learn to walk: how often do they fall down? Hundreds of times each day, before they can finally take their first step and even then, it's always only a tiny little step they start with. They will leverage on the success of that first little, shaky step to take a second one and then a third one. They won't feel steady for a long time, but the thought of giving up never even crosses their mind. That's because babies only live in the present. They don't obsess with what went wrong yesterday, they're too focused on having fun today.

The process of learning to walk for them is not some hurdle they're enduring: it's a fun and exciting process they're present with and making the most of. They're almost not thinking about the end goal, they're just having fun each step of the way (literally) and once they get going, they simply can't stop.

As much as possible, embrace and enjoy each step. Even the falls. Everything has its place and purpose. Everything is teaching you something you need to learn to progress so notice and celebrate every little improvement, embrace and leverage on every little challenge. Know that what you learn along the way is profoundly more important than some end goal you're trying to achieve and if you learn to embrace the journey, you truly will get further and faster than you could have ever imagined.

CHAPTER 7

Overcoming Hurdles

This section is actually designed as a mini motivational section that you can come back to time and time again to reaffirm your commitment, regain inspiration, overcome periods of difficulties and come back to yourself and your journey. Of course you can read the whole book as often as needed, even once a month to begin with. If you feel time pressed however and just need a quick pick-me-up to fire you up, read the following chapters and you'll find the motivation and inspiration to keep going.

After all is said and done, I'd like to remind you of a few things that are very important and will never stop being relevant and useful no matter how far you are on the journey to your most fit, healthy and confident self.

Firstly please remember that progress is not linear. You're not gonna get progressively better and better without any setbacks. Setbacks are inevitable. They are a fundamental part of life. They're designed to teach us something and can generally be used to propel us forward with renewed determination and focus.

They don't mean we're a failure. They don't necessarily mean the method is failing us, although in some instances, they may be pointing us in a slightly different direction.

If you learn to recognize them with curiosity, rather than judgement you'll become better and better at using them in a positive way.

The road to success is made of tiny little moments of ups and downs but as long as you're headed in the right direction and don't allow a difficulty to take you off your chosen path, you will get there for sure. The important thing is not to use any difficulty as an excuse for giving up. The only way you're NOT gonna get to your goals is if you give up.

Stay with it. If something doesn't work for you even after several attempts, than maybe that specific habit, food, exercise routine is not the right one for you so try something different. Just because it worked for someone else it doesn't mean it's the right thing for you also. We're all different. What you don't want to do is use it as an excuse to reinforce a past negative belief about how " You're just not meant to be fit and heathy. It's not for you. You don't care about it enough. It's not in your genes. You don't know what you're doing. You just can't change" and on and on down the list of limiting beliefs that don't serve you well.

So be prepared: you're gonna get it wrong at some point and in some way. More than once. It's gonna happen. Even if you hire the best professional on the market because guess what, they won't be with you 24/7 for 1-3 solid years. So there will be times when you make a decision that you'll regret and that's fine. Get back on track AS SOON AS POSSIBLE. Don't fall down the "oh no, I've blown it" trap which leads to us giving up.

Learn what you're meant to be learning, tweak what you're meant to be tweaking and get back at it with renewed passion and determination. Please trust me when I say that it is SO worth it in the end.

The second thing I'd like to remind you of is that you're never going to be done with this. Ever. Yes, you read that right. You will never be done. The journey to your most fit, healthy and confident self is the journey of a lifetime. There is no end to it. It will continue for as long as you live or as long as you give up on yourself. I've made a quiet yet strong commitment to myself that I will NEVER give up on myself. Therefore I will never stop growing, evolving, improving and bettering my health and wellbeing.

Sure, there will be times when you'll simply maintain the results of a period of hard work and will simply be following a routine that works for you. Then there will be times when you'll get tested and perhaps take a few steps back and will have to go through a bit of a sprint to get back on track. Then there will be times when something that worked for you for years will stop working and you'll have to investigate the best move forward. You get the message.

As long as you keep reminding yourself of the importance of not giving up on your health and wellbeing, you'll continue to improve, grow and progress in whichever way works best for you and at whatever pace you are meant to.

The most important thing is to not give up because you know what they say: the moment you stop growing, you'll start dying.

Become Greater Than Your Environment

Today is July 31st 2019: it's the first of our mini four day break in Sicily. We've rented a little room by the most beautiful beach on the island to take a well-deserved short break after hosting a super successful luxury wellness retreat on Mount Etna. It was a beautiful experience, yet quite tiring as we worked relentlessly to make sure that all our guests' needs were met 24/7, for 5 days. It went super well and everyone wants to come back next year: I was feeling tired yet elated, joyful, satisfied and fulfilled. Now I feel overwhelmed, sad and guilty.

It all changed in a matter of minutes. About 30 to be precise. As long as that phone call with my father. It just never fails. I'm not blaming him in any way: he doesn't know what he's doing and doesn't know any different. My dad was diagnosed with bipolar disorder when I was only 8 years old and has since progressively gotten worse and worse. It remains the most challenging experience of my entire life. I even produced and co-directed a documentary on my family's experience called "Tale Padre". I am lucky enough to have overcome the hurdles of my childhood and turned them mostly into opportunities for growth and self-development.

Most days, I am even minded and can approach matters concerning my father and my family in a logical and balanced way. For some reason however, this becomes much harder when I am in physical proximity to him: whenever I'm back in Italy, I notice I get more easily dragged into the mud of his psychotic and dysfunctional behaviors and have to work much harder at staying in touch with myself. With my core. I get catapulted back to the person I was before I left Italy, 14 long years ago. The guilt I grew up with (the guilt of simply being alive), starts overtaking me and before I know it, I lose prospective of all the good and only notice the bad.

That's what's happening right now, after a mere 30 minutes phone call with him who doesn't know how not to dump all his paranoia, anxiety and fear on those around him. And just like that, I spend two solid hours of my precious 4 days break (the first holiday this year and possibly the last until Christmas) crying my eyes out and unable to leave my bed. I am then finally able to pull myself together and head to the beach with my very patient husband who is gently reminding me to breath and "come back to myself" but even at the beach I find it hard to switch my mind off the negative thought patterns that are now running out of control. At this point, I've wasted a solid 4 hours of my precious and well deserved break.

That's when it finally hits me: I know better now! I've practiced how to come back from this often but it's harder when I'm here because everything reminds my mind and body of my past. It's really that simple. There are way more triggers to remind me of the difficult times so my brain finds it harder to come back to the present moment.

I then remember that I do carry with me a positive trigger that I know can make it all better: I plug my headphones into my iPhone and turn on a one hour guided meditation. I am sitting on a lounge chair, under the umbrella, in the most crowded beach there is, at the peak of Sicilian summer so it takes a little bit longer than usual to get lost into the words and detach myself from my surroundings but about half way through, I manage and by the time the meditation is over, I'm back to my balanced and even minded self.

Back in the days, that phone call would have spoiled my entire holiday and possibly a few days after that too. Today, it only took four hours. Next year it may take two hours. One day it will take minutes, if that.

When your environment does not support your greatest goals and aspirations, you've got to become greater than your environment; this does not happen spontaneously and takes practice. Daily practice. The more rooted you are in your daily practices of mindfulness, the less affected you'll be by the inevitable storms that life will bring your way. If you wait for your life to get easier before you learn how to take better care of yourself, you'll be waiting a long time. Life doesn't get easier, you simply get stronger and when you're stronger and more rooted, it takes way more to upset you.

I haven't yet mastered the art of not being affected by certain triggers in my environment: I have however developed techniques and methodologies to shorten the gap between an upsetting instance and me regaining my composure. Every year, the gap gets shorter. Every year I practice more, not less, of the self-care techniques that I know bring me back to my best self and keep me grounded and rooted into positive feelings, thoughts, vibrations.

You can become greater than your environment and when that happens, you'll find that you'll start being able to affect IT more than it affects YOU. Not by deliberately trying though because your efforts will still only go towards your own self-care above all else.

Don't wait for things to change around you. Change YOU. Better YOU. Learn to take the best possible care of yourself now and that will have the most profound, positive impact on your entire life in ways that go beyond your greatest expectations.

That time is NOW. If you're waiting for a sign from the universe, THIS IS IT. Don't settled for a miserable life. Pain is not natural. Don't wait for things to get easier, they may never do. Take one small new step in the direction to your most fit, healthy and confident self NOW and never look back. You have nothing to lose and everything to gain. Everyone will benefit from it. Your life will get better. The life of those around you will get better.

Self-care is not an option, it is your greatest responsibility because if you don't take care of yourself, soon enough, someone will have to take care of you. So Be Selfish. Be Selfless. Play Big. Most importantly, start NOW.

Seven Harsh Truths Of Long Lasting Weight Loss

My relationship with food and eating hasn't always been plain sailing: quite the opposite in fact. Food was my drug of choice growing up and my preferred tool to cope with the trauma of growing up with a mentally ill father. I'm grateful though, not only because I could have easily chosen a WAY more destructive and debilitation coping mechanism, but also because those challenges taught me SO much of what I know now. By really understanding the subtle dynamics of what I call the "psychology of eating" I am able to help our clients identify the root causes of their unbalances with food which is a FUNDAMENTAL step to achieving long lasting results. Here's the thing, you can eat all the "right" foods and know everything there is to know about healthier choices, calories, macro-nutrients etc. but if you don't investigate and improve how you eat and why, you will struggle to find peace and effortlessly maintain a healthy weight. Most of us know a lot about how we could improve our diets to get positive results: why is it so hard to make the necessary changes then? The answer lies precisely in your very unique "psychology of eating".

Having said all that, there are some harsh and universals truths around eating and weight-loss that I've found apply to everyone's journey to some extent, and will certainly help you make the shift in perspective that's needed to improve. I've come to identify these in my work with hundreds of busy and time pressed professionals all around the world and I truly believe you will get value and insights that you can implement right away.

So here they come: the 7 harsh truths of long lasting weight-loss:

1. **Diets DON'T work:** fact! Most of us have been on a diet
at some point or another in our lives: in fact I would be
inclined to guess that most of us have been on a diet
more than once in our lives. You may even be on a diet
RIGHT NOW! But how many times can we do the
same thing, hoping to achieve a different outcome?
If diets worked, we wouldn't put the weight back on (and
then some) in less than half the time it took to lose it.
Think about every diet you have ever done in your life:
how much time, money and effort did you invest?
How long did the results last? Dieting is inherently
flawed because it is based around the faulty principle that
we can follow a strict regimen for a set amount of time
until we get the intended result, and then maintain said
results even after the diet is over. Or even worse, we fool
ourselves to think that the only way to have a lean and
healthy body is by being on a diet for the rest of our life!
I mean, seriously! The only way to achieve real and long
lasting results is by making small, incremental improvements and give yourself enough time to embed these in
your routine for good until you simply won't know
another way of eating. It won't be something that you're
doing just to lose a few pounds. It will be your routine
and will come second nature to you. Any change that is
not sustainable for the rest of your life, is not healthy
change and whatever results you may get from it are
NOT yours for the rest of your life. The sooner you come
to realize and accept this hard fact, the sooner you'll
be able to then STOP wasting time, energy and money
on what doesn't work and start focusing on what will.
This principle also applies to things such as detoxes, juice
cleanse and any other very extreme and calorie deficient
regimen with a healthy spin around it. I'm not saying

that there is NO point in doing a detox or juice cleanse but those are DEFINITELY not modalities that should be used to achieve long term weight-loss on their own; they should only ever be a part of a greater and wholistic plan of action which ultimately revolves around sustainable habits that can be maintained forever.

2. **There is no "magic pill" (or potion, or herb):** in my mind this is really so obvious that it shouldn't require mentioning, however I am constantly surprised to meet smart, successful individuals in my daily practice who still want to believe in some magic pill, supplement, herb or potion which will deliver the promised results without nasty side effects or, most importantly, without needing to make any changes to what they eat and how they eat it. This is probably one of the most debilitating side effects of chronic, long term dieting: we end up so disempowered and delusional from the tiring rollercoaster of diet on/diet off that in the end our only hope is to believe in some miracle product which will rescue us from the oblivion. Of course, such a product DOES NOT exist. Generally, the secret to profound results does not lie in anything that you're currently missing from your diet, it's more likely to be the many things that should be missing from it. I appreciate that the notion of "eliminating" foods from one's diet can spark feelings of deprivation, but that's only the case if this is not done in a sensible and systematic way (which is how most commercial diets do it). That's why I have devised an approach which I call "crowding out". By putting the emphasis on increasing the amount of heath promoting foods in our diets, we naturally leave less room for the

foods that don't support our goals, without going hungry (bad news) or feeling deprived (really bad news).

3. **There is NO real way of eating crap and still being healthy and slim:** this is essentially how most fad diets came about. The market was simply looking to give people what they wanted and apparently what they wanted was a way to eat bacon, butter and steaks but still lose weight. This is a big topic that's really hard to condense and the reason why fad diets have gained traction is because they do generate short to medium term results. Especially with people who were eating a diet mainly consisting of junk food: the truth is that any improvement from a junk food diet will bring forth positive results. The same can be said for systems such as Weight Watchers or any calorie restricting program; these resolve around the principle that to lose weight, one must simply cut down on the calories consumed each day. The problem with this approach is that not all calories are created equal: 100 kcal of cake will have a profoundly different effect on the body than 100 kcal of beans or broccoli. If you go from consuming 5,000 kcal a day to consuming 2,500 you WILL lose weight BUT, and this is a KEY difference, if you're not eating enough of the foods with highest nutrient density, long lasting results will continue to escape you. In order to function optimally, the body doesn't just need a minimum amount of calories each day but also and most importantly, it needs essential macro and micro nutrients and guess what? If you're not getting enough nutrients, much like when you don't get enough calories, you will continuously feel ravenous or weak, or lack energy even as you get leaner. I always remind our shifters that in most cases, calorie counting is simply distracting

and deceiving. The focus should be on eating PLENTY of nutrient dense foods such as vegetables, fruit, wholegrain and legumes, and eating those without limits until we feel satisfied and full. That's the only monitoring ever required for effortless and long lasting result.

4. **You can't outrun a bad diet:** now this is a big one that we see reoccurring time and again especially in very active individuals who love sport. Don't get me wrong, fitness is a fundamental pillar of wholistic wellbeing and long lasting weight-loss however, no amount of fitness will ever undo the negative effects of a bad diet. You can run a marathon a day, lift weights 4 times a week, do Hot Yoga until you melt but if you still eat crap, your optimum level of wellbeing will continue to escape you. You may even go as far as achieving your ideal body on the outside, but you just will not be healthy from the inside out, which is the only real way of being healthy. This is what confuses lots of people and the reason why even apparently healthy individuals can be struck by chronic diseases such as diabetes, heart disease and cancer. Looking fit and lean shouldn't be the main outcome of your wellness journey: being truly and holistically healthy from the inside out should be the outcome and looking fit and lean is just a welcome side effect of that. If you shift your perspective from simply wanting to lose weight, to wanting to achieve genuine and permanent health and wellbeing, you will feel WAY more profoundly motivated and driven, you will make healthier and smarter choices along the way AND you will achieve greater results than you even thought possible. When all we care about is losing a few pounds, we enter a dangerous mindset of "I will do anything to just lose the weight" and our

judgment will be clouded. That's when we start looking for unhealthy short-cuts and miracle solutions. Instead, when we look at ourselves as a whole, our life as a whole and our health and wellbeing as the number one priority, we give much more importance to the things that matter most. From that perspective then, you won't exercise just so that you can eat junk or drink too much without putting weight on: you will exercise because you want to take the best possible care of the most important possession in your life. Your body!

5. **Only you choose what to put in your mouth:** Nobody can MAKE you, nothing can TEMPT you if you don't want to be tempted, no smell can be TOO alluring or circumstance too TRICKY to navigate. Those are all excuses, plain and simple! The choice is and forever remains yours in the end. Taking full responsibility for your life and your choices is a fundamental step in achieving anything in life, but in particular, in making the improvements needed to lose weight and get healthy once and for all. I know those road blocks sometimes really feel like deal breakers but I will tell you with absolute certainty that they only are if you allow them to be. I'm not saying this to make you feel bad or guilty: quite the opposite. I'm saying this to put the power back firmly in your hands where it belongs. I often use this simple technique with our shifters, whenever they talk about an aunt forcing an unwanted celebration meal down their throat or a colleague making them eat birthday cake by giving them the evil eye. I simply then ask them this question "what would you have done if they were offering you a food that you're terribly allergic to and that would make you sick and send you to hospital?" My guess is that you

would politely decline without even a second thought: it wouldn't be a struggle to say no. You wouldn't have a back and forth with yourself as to whether you should accept and then live with the consequences. You also (and this is the MOST important detail) wouldn't feel BAD about not accepting a food that you know is bad for you. It really wouldn't matter what your aunt or colleague said or did: the answer would be a firm, resolute and non-conditional "NO". So if you're really committed to your journey, if you're really present and aware of why you're choosing to avoid certain foods, if you're non-conditional about the fact your health and wellbeing are the most important thing in your life, nothing, nobody, no event or circumstance will ever be too difficult for you to navigate. It's that simple (although simple doesn't always mean easy).

6. **All taste is acquired besides from breast milk:** you CAN learn to enjoy simpler food if you choose to. Taste is not absolute, it is not set in stone, it is not binding and most importantly it is NOT in charge of your wellness journey. Guess who's in charge? That's right, you are. Letting taste dictate your choices is a little bit like allowing a toddler to run your household: they will most definitely fail you but not because they want to, simply because they don't know any better. Don't get me wrong here: I'm not an advocate of boring and tasteless food that you don't enjoy. Enjoying the journey and pleasures in life is a fundamental part of a healthy and balanced routine but these joys should NEVER come at the detriment of your health. In fact, learning to enjoy simpler pleasures in life will make a huge difference not only to your weight-loss journey but your life as a whole. In many

cases in fact, our taste buds have actually been hijacked by the prolonged consumption of processed foods high in fat, sugar and salt so you've effectively lost the taste for the foods that we're meant to be eating. Remember that you can easily become used to and even learn to enjoy something that's actually not good for you if it stimulates your dopamine centers in a certain way: that's ultimately how cigarettes, alcohol and drugs work. Think of when you were little: I'm sure you can come up with at least a handful of items that you really disliked when you first tried them but you now love. Retraining your taste buds is not only possible, it's necessary to achieve permanent results: it should be done in a smart and systematic way to make the process as effortless as possible but it can't be avoided. The more you embrace and enjoy trying new, healthier foods or going back to more wholesome eating habits, the higher (and faster) your rate of success. There's a reason why the kings and queens of the world used to die prematurely from chronic diseases that were unknown to the peasants: the goal is to live like kings and queens but eat like peasants so that we can have the best of both worlds!

7. **It takes longer than you think:** to bring forth permanent and profound improvements so you better learn to love and embrace the process. The good news is: if you go about it the heathy and wholistic way, once you get the results they're yours for good. There will be no slipping back to the old ways. You will never be unable to resist something you know is not conducive to your goals and new lifestyle anymore. All those foods will completely lose any hold over you. You will stop craving them and even considering them "edible food at all". Trust me when

I say that I really don't have to work very hard at eating healthy, AT ALL. It is NOT a matter of willpower, I don't have to work hard to resist the abundance of junk food available to us every day. There is no tug of war going on in my life. I actually crave my healthy meals, in fact that's all I can think of eating most days. Once or twice a week I eat out and would go for so something more processed and rich than anything I ever cook at home: for sure I enjoy those moments but I never ever crave them more than occasionally. I don't just LOVE the healthy foods I eat routinely, I also and most importantly LOVE how they make me feel. I'm very present to how my body responds to food, so the idea of eating something that makes me feel sluggish, stuffed, bloated and heavy is actually not appealing at all most days. And if you're thinking that I'm special or I'm different or I'm making this up, I promise you that I am not. This state is available to ANY human being on the planet: it doesn't happen overnight and it does take some work and effort especially in the initial stages but once established, it is yours for life. In fact I would go as far as saying that it should be your ultimate objective. Your body wants to be healthy, lean and fit: any state other than that is NOT its natural state. Look around in nature: do you see any other mammals struggling with obesity and food related chronic diseases (other than the poor domesticated cats and dogs WE feed)? Your body is not failing you, ever. The opposite is true in fact: you're failing to take care of it the way it needs to be but the moment you recognize and make the relevant adjustments you'll discover that it is your greatest ally in life and wants nothing more than for you to have a glorious, happy and fulfilled life for as long as possible.

10 Tips For Holidays And Special Occasions

Christmas (or any other holiday for that matter) is certainly a cherished time for most people: a time of joyous celebration with family and friends. A time to take a break from our daily routines, enjoy some (often long overdue) time off and embrace traditions we've known and looked forward to since we were little. For many years however, I was never fully capable of truly enjoying this time of the year without also experiencing some conflicting and even unpleasant emotions. The thing is, I like my routines, especially around food and eating; so for a long time, I struggled to find a way to enjoy this festive period whilst also staying grounded in my fitness, nutrition and wellbeing needs.

As previously mentioned, food and nutrition were not always easy subjects for me. It took me years however to establish healthy and balanced routines around eating and that is why for years I really struggled during the holiday period.

Don't get me wrong, I LOVE a treat and an extravagant meal much like any other person out there however, this time of the year takes indulgence to a whole new level! I know that within the context of daily healthy eating Monday through Friday, a blow out on Saturday night is not going to affect me negatively. In fact I've made such occurrences a fundamental part of my routine and I really look forward to it when it comes. I do also always look forward to going back to my healthier and cleaner meals on Sunday.

Christmas is different though: where I'm from in Sicily, we start eating on Christmas eve and hardly take a break until January 2nd! That can be a solid 8 days of consecutive feasts and let me tell you, that'll put a dent into anyone's wellbeing, no matter how fit and healthy they are! So how do you navigate this time without completely losing it and getting to January feeling like you've set yourself back a few months? It took me years to figure this out but finally, I've come up with a list of 10 top tips that really works for me. They may not ALL apply to you but I'm sure MANY of them will and I truly hope you can find some inspiration and motivation to make it through this time of the year feeling empowered and in control while still enjoying it.

So here it goes: top 10 wellness tips for a VERY merry Christmas:

1. Set some non-negotiable boundaries and stick to them NO MATTER WHAT: They don't have to be many nor do they have to be really strict. Keep them real but also constructive and then stick to them. No matter what. This will make you feel more confident, certain and happy with yourself.

2. Write your non-negotiable rules down: just thinking about them is not enough. Pen on paper is a must as it works your neuron-pathways in a different way to help you really engrain the ideas in your consciousness PLUS this will help with tip #3.

3. Read your non-negotiable rules every day: a daily reminder of your own commitments to your wellbeing can make ALL the difference and will prevent you from losing track. Your mind needs training so by reading these guidelines every day you will prevent slip ups that may turn into an "all out" scenario.

4. Share your non-negotiable rules openly: I don't mean stopping people at the supermarket to tell them all about why you don't eat chocolate before 5pm. Nor do I mean lecturing your friends and families on all your

commitment but if the occasion arises, be honest and open. If your aunt offers you something you are committed to not eating, drinking or doing at that moment in time, feel free to tell her about your non-negotiable boundaries, why you've come up with them and how they help you stay on track. You never know, you may just inspire someone to improve their own approach. As long as your stance is non-judgmental and non-preachy, it will go a LONG way.

5. Drink water: lots of it. Every. Single. Day. Otherwise you'll increase the risk of feeling sluggish, bloated and not energized. Not to mention drinking water helps to flush out any extra toxins, keeps your bowel movements regular AND prevents you from over-eating (remember that sometimes we think we're hungry when in fact we're just thirsty).

6. Eat raw fruit EVERY SINGLE DAY. The more fiber you eat, the better. This is true at any time of the year but especially when you're eating more elaborate foods than usual. This will also make sure you're getting plenty of vitamins and minerals, not just empty calories from chocolates and cookies. Plus a piece of fruit or a raw veggie can cleanse the pallet AND will make you feel very good about yourself!

7. Eat raw vegetables EVERY SINGLE DAY. See above!

8. Move your body EVERY SINGLE DAY. DISCLAIMER: this does NOT have to mean going to the gym. I completely appreciate that you may want or need to take a break from your traditional fitness routine but if you can find a way to stay active every single day, you'll feel SO much better for it, not just physically but also, and most importantly, emotionally. You can dance to your

favorite christmas tunes, go for a walk in nature or play active games with the kids in the house. Anything will do and if it's fun, even better!

9. Spend some time alone, even just a few minutes, EVERY SINGLE DAY. As much as we (mostly) enjoy reconnecting with family and friends, it can get a bit overwhelming to jump from one social engagement to the next for a solid week or more. Make sure you make time for silence and solitude daily. Even if it's just a few minutes. This will make you feel more grounded and prevent possible burnout and feelings of resentment.

10. Remember it's only once a year so after all is said and done, make sure you have fun and truly cherish every single moment you spend with your loved ones.

Handling Peer Pressure

This is a sticky subject which comes up in our conversations with our shifters time and again, especially in relations to nutrition. Making the shift towards healthier habits is hard enough as it is, but can be made even harder by those around us who, without even trying to, may come across as unsupportive of our goals and therefore add another layer of challenge.

The ideal case scenario would obviously be to have conversations with those who are closest to us so that you can get them onboard and not have to continuously deal with confrontation that may hinder our progress by make you doubt and question yourself. Anybody you live with should be made aware of your goals and aspirations so that you can build a support system that can make all the difference along the way. If you can, you may even want to enroll them into keeping you accountable during challenging moments and spurring you on when needed.

Always remember that human beings are not naturally self-motivated and we give our best when our accountability is outsourced, and we have someone outside of ourselves to motivate and inspire us, but also to show us our blind spots which we could never see on our own. That's why hiring a coach can make all the difference on your journey. If you can find someone that not only has plenty of experience in working with individuals as yourself, but also most importantly who inspires and motivates you, who speaks to your heart and whose message resonates with you, you will boost your success rate immensely and you will find it one of the greatest investments you'll ever make.

There are some instances however when it may not be possible to get the support of those around us: that's totally ok and should not be used as an excuse to not make the improvements we know we need to make. If somebody you live with doesn't see eye to eye with the changes you're implementing, it can be useful to simply agree to disagree rather than continuously embark on confronting conversations that may just drain your energy and distract you from what you should actually be focusing on.

Having to constantly defend your choices can ultimately have a negative impact on your motivation so I would highly discourage it. It would be much better to find a peaceful agreement whereby, even though said person doesn't agree with your choices, they respect them by not continually talk about them negatively. You can then look for the encouragement and support you need elsewhere.

Trying to convince somebody else should not be your goal or focus. You should only focus on your own journey and lead by example, which may just eventually inspire change in those around you, but that should in no way be your main aim.

You can't spark change in someone who's not ready to change or who doesn't see anything wrong with their life and habits: this only generally results in them getting defensive and closing themselves off to the possibility of self-improvement even further. The best way to facilitate change in others is to lead by example and be the change you want to see; so by focusing on your life only, you will end up having a far greater positive influence than if you turn into a preacher and tell everyone what they should be doing and why.

This approach is even more useful if the unsupportive friend or family member is not actually that close to you (i.e. you don't live with them and don't see them more than once a week):

do everything you can to maintain a neutral stance and avoid going any deep into the whats and whys. The high road is the answer. If they offer you a food item you've chosen not to eat for now, you can say things like "I've found it doesn't make me feel good so thank you, but no thank you" or "my doctor has suggested I avoid this for now". Anything that won't confront them directly, and won't require a great deal of explanation, is the best answer.

If you're going to a dinner party and you know the host won't cook anything that will work for you or you don't want to impose by specifying your eating preferences, you could:

- eat before you go and only have very little of the healthiest options on offer there (you can say you're not feeling too hungry as you made the silly mistake of having a late snack. Or you can say your stomach has been upset and you don't want to overdo it). You can shift the focus to the company and catching up with your friends more than the food.
- bring along something you can eat and in enough quantities for everyone to try too
- join them only for drinks after dinner or before

If you generally go out with friends to a restaurant you know is not particularly healthy, you could:

- suggest a new place that has a variety you know will work for all of you
- call the regular restaurant to see if they can accommodate your requirements
- again, eat before you go and only have a small starter.

If there's a will, there's a way and there are plenty of solutions for all kind of circumstances so that you don't have to choose between having fun and being your best self. After all how much fun is there in doing something you know will make you feel bad for a very long time?

Afterword

I hope you enjoyed reading this book as much as I enjoyed writing it. I hope it spoke to your heart as much as your mind because let's be frank, NO intelligence is more powerful than that of your heart. Now is time to align your heart, mind and feet and take MASSIVE action in the direction to your most fit, healthy and confident self.

Please be aware, this is not the end, it's merely the beginning. The ideas and principles I've shared with you in this book are carefully designed to #sparktheshift to your greatest self yet, Don't forget, it can take minutes or hours to spark the shift but it takes months or years to **#maketheshift**

In finishing this book, you have already achieved more than many people do,so well done for that. Celebrate this accomplishment and leverage your success to motivate you further: after all, your work is just beginning.

You now have plenty of tools to act upon and implement in your everyday life with determination, consistency and the drive that such important matters require. Treat your health and wellbeing as if it were the most important matter in your life and it will never become a "matter of urgency".

Don't EVER give up on yourself. Keep coming back to the chapters that spoke to you most, Read them multiple times to re-ignite the spark as often as needed. Don't hesitate to ask for help and don't be too proud to outsource your accountability. Do what you have to do and do it NOW. There is no better time.

Life is too precious and short to live it like anything other than your very best self.

With love, Serena

Acknowledgements

Although it only took me three months to write, this book is actually 35 years in the making. It is the fruit of my entire life's experiences and work. Everything I have been through, all my jobs, training, relationships and travels have profoundly contributed to its content: I am so grateful for it all.

I would love to thank every single person who has crossed my path but that may be tricky so, for the sake of time and paper, I will limit myself.

I'd like to start by thanking every single one of our shifters (clients): present, past and future. I am humbled and grateful that you have chosen us to facilitate your transformation and entrusted us with the health and wellbeing of the most important person in your life. From the bottom of my heart, I thank you.

I did not believe in soul mates until I met mine: Eugene Sabala. You are a greater life (and business) partner than I ever dared to dream of. I thank the Universe for reuniting us in the life and many more to come.

I'd like to thank my sister Alice, who is an endless source of wisdom, inspiration, motivation and comfort. I just couldn't imagine my life without our unbreakable bond.

To my parents, who have truly (and literally) made me who I am: I could not have asked for better guidance. Truly. You've taught me every single most important lesson in this life. Your unconditional love and support has given me the courage to pursue my dreams. Thank you.

I'd like to thank my entire extended family but in particular my uncles Rino and Vito, my auntie Graziella, their spouses and children and my grandma Rina: your help during difficult times has been SO invaluable and has allowed me to create a better life for myself than I would have otherwise been able to.

To my dearest friends in Italy, England and the US (you know who you are!): your support and encouragement remain invaluable every single day of my life. Thank you.

To my yoga tribe: a selection of remarkable individuals, scattered all over the world, whose friendship enriches my life regardless of how often we get to meet and spend time together. Thank you.

To my business tribe: I couldn't ask for better mentors, coaches, business partners and accountability buddies. Every single one of you inspires me to keep going and reach higher. Thank you.

Next Steps

Here are more resources you can use to leverage on the momentum you've built and continue to #maketheshift

The Mind-Body Confidence Score card

This is a completely FREE tool we have developed to help you score your current level of development across the three pillars of wellbeing (Focus, Food, Fitness): It takes roughly 5 minutes to complete and will allow you to identify the areas with most room for improvements. Answer the questions and check your inbox for a comprehensive and bespoke PDF report including your scores and effective tips to start making improvements.

http://www.wholeshiftwellness.com/scorecard/

Complimentary PDF reports

As a thank you for reading this book, we'd like to share with you some reports which are designed to complement the contents of this book. These are:

1. "7 Mistakes": a report which details the 7 most common mistakes we see busy professionals make when trying to improve their health and wellbeing and how to prevent them.

   https://mailchi.mp/dd15b33cf12f/freepdf7mistakes

2. "7 days to #sparktheshift": a comprehensive e-book containing Focus, Food and Fitness tips for an entire week. It includes recipes with pictures and a detailed workout plan with photo-instructions to help you get started on the road to your most fit, healthy and confident self.

   email us on:
   info@wholeshiftwellness.com (subject: e-book)

Events

If you live in London and would like to meet us in person, you can join us for one of our super informative boardroom events. We host these at convenient central locations in the City.

Visit our events page on Facebook for more information.

https://www.facebook.com/wholeshiftwellness/events

And if you'd like to #sparktheshift in the most amazing location, whilst also relaxing, sunbathing, discovering the Italian countryside and bonding with like-minded individuals, you may want to join us for one of our luxury wellness retreats in Sicily.

https://www.wholeshiftwellness.com/retreat/

Strategy Session

If you'd like to find out more about our Shifts and how we transform the health and wellbeing of time pressed professionals, you can schedule a complimentary 45 minutes strategy session with Serena in person or via video call. Subject to availability.

email us on:
info@wholeshiftwellness.com (subject: strategy session)

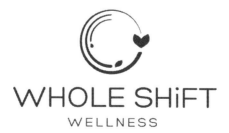

About The Author

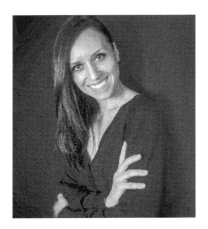

Serena Sabala

Serena is a Certified Plant Based Nutrition Consultant, Yoga Teacher and Fitness Trainer who has studied nutrition for over ten years and has a unique, wholistic approach to health and wellness.

When she was only 8 years old her father, a very successful and busy entrepreneur, got really sick: unfortunately he didn't have the tools to take care of his own wellbeing and therefore crumbled under the pressure of owning a multi-million euros business.

This led to him losing everything he had worked so hard for, which had huge consequences for him and the whole family.

As a result of her childhood experiences, Serena has developed an interest in wellbeing practices which started at a very young age.

Today, together with her husband Eugene, she runs Whole Shift Wellness: a coaching company specialised in bespoke programs for time pressed professionals. Their combined experience spans over 20+ years and has allowed them to work with more than 500 professionals across 5 countries. Together, they passionately apply their proven methodology to transform the health and wellbeing of leaders from around the world who want to be strong, fit, healthy and satisfied, and who aspire to continue having a positive impact within their organizations and the communities around them.

Serena is also very passionate about bringing wellness to the workplace, since many people spend most of their waking hours at work: she believes that "employees who are cared for, care more" and that companies who put the wellbeing of their employees at the forefront of what they do, are more successful than average.

Printed in Poland
by Amazon Fulfillment
Poland Sp. z o.o., Wrocław

53883822R00099